WHAT PEOPLE ARE SAYING

This honest, humorous and helpful devotional *must-read for anyone facing medical issues or servin* *personal stories, advice and prayers will get you through any of life's challenges!*

~ Susan M. Heim, *Chicken Soup for the Soul* editor

As a Registered Nurse, I encounter all types of patients and at many different stages of life. The ones that appear to fair the best are those who have a strong faith in Christ, a willingness to learn and be an active participant in their current health issues and use humor to help fight the fear that comes along with illness. Loretta Schoen's Surviving Medical Mayhem helps the reader do just that. With humor and strong messages of faith, she arms the reader with the tools necessary in surviving todays medical industry.

~ Kimberly Brown, RN, BSN

I'm genuinely a healthy person and tend to lament even a minor cold. As I get older I know it won't be the case... All patch, patch, patch after 50! God has a plan and your book reminded me to take it all in stride, with an Erma Bombeck sense of humor.

~Karin L. Veatch, Wealth Advisor, Private Bank, J.P. Morgan

Theologian Dallas Willard said we will never really understand God until we understand that God is the most joyful being in the universe. Loretta Schoen gets that. Her book is filled with the kind of joy-in-the-face-of-adversity that can only come from a lifelong relationship with a loving and joyful God. Sandy and I laughed out loud as we read this wonderful book by our friend Loretta. Her deep faith in a loving and joyful God shines through every story. During our 40 years of ministry we often won-

dered how people who don't know God make it through the kind of crises that Loretta navigates with faith, courage and joy.

~Pastor Ken & Sandy Roughton, United Methodist Ministry Team

Thank you for sharing your book. You truly have a gift for writing. The blend of a life riddled with challenges, humor and GOD!! What else could a Christian ask for in a book. I believe this book will help anyone going through medical challenges. This book will give them some tools to work with, Bible quotes to reflect on and hope that they too can make it through with strength and humor.

~ Dr. Theresa K. Goebel D.O, Cornerstone Family Practice

What an inspirational message Loretta Schoen has to offer. This book has a great message for anyone dealing with health or medical issues, a real inspirational support. Well done Loretta!

~ Christopher B. Warren, CLU, ChFC, "Your Personal CFO," Partner

Nearly everyone has had a brush with today's medical system, which often fixes bodies without paying much attention to the people inside those bodies—leaving us, as Loretta D. Schoen puts it, fine (Frightened, Insecure, Neurotic, Exhausted). Her book Surviving Medical Mayhem: Laughing When it Hurts is a wonderful response to this problem, giving us concrete advice on how we can take steps to become fine (Faith-filled, Involved, knowledgeable, and Experienced).

P.S.: It's also an interesting and remarkably funny read.

~Salvatore Basile, author of *Fifth Avenue Famous and COOL: How Air Conditioning Changed Everything*

Surviving Medical Mayhem

Laughing When It Hurts

Surviving Medical Mayhem

Laughing When It Hurts

Loretta D. Schoen

Surviving Medical Mayhem: Laughing When It Hurts
by Loretta D. Schoen

Published by HigherLife Development Services, Inc.
PO Box 623307
Oviedo, Florida 32762
(407) 563-4806
www.ahigherlife.com

ISBN 978-0-9989773-9-3

First Edition
13 14 15 16 17 —12 11 10 9 8 7 6 5
Printed in the United States of America

ACKNOWLEDGMENTS

I would like to thank God for His presence and grace throughout my life. He has never wavered in His constant love and has guided me through every dark corridor. He has provided me with signs to know that He is present and that I am ultimately in *His* care. He truly has been my lifeline when I could see no other.

I wish to thank many health-care professionals. I wrote *Surviving Medical Mayhem* in part because of the frustration I felt in the managed health-care system that manifested itself in poor health care and because of changes in the medical-care system caused, in part, by the loss of excellent professionals. However, many professionals continue to provide excellence and quality care to the patients as individuals, not as numbers, dollars, and insurance reimbursement opportunities.

Thanks go to Dr. Frank Cirisano for his personal care that allowed me to formulate the idea, and to Dr. Elizabeth McKeen, who encouraged me to work on this project and showed me what a good Christian physician and practice is like. I would be remiss if I did not include the wonderful nurses, technicians, and other health-care professionals who have cared for my family and me. Their true love and compassion prompted my desire to share what I have learned about empowering the patient.

I must thank my daughter, Francesca, who not only read and edited each story initially but spurred me on with her faith and support in this project. Her belief in this project and in *me* motivated me to continue when I wanted to walk away and get a "real" job. Thank you, Peanut, for teaching me as much as I have taught you, and maybe more!

And finally, but foremost, to my husband, Thad: thank you for your patience, love, and support for me during what I call my "panda moments." There were times when I was like a panda stomping about in frustration without any bamboo to feed on and generally creating pandemonium along my path. Without you and our life together, I would never have created *Surviving Medical Mayhem*. Thank you for encouraging me in spite of myself.

And to those of you who have purchased this book: thank you for allowing me to give back some of what I have received.

With sincerity and prayers for peace and wellness,

Loretta Schoen

CONTENTS

PREFACE

From the time I was a little girl, I dreamed of being a writer. A family friend was a famous writer, and after sharing my dream with her, she told me that writers write what they know. At the time, I thought, "I don't know much about anything, God. What shall I write about?" But the wonderful thing about life and our Father in heaven is that He answers prayers. We may not understand His ways, but He always answers the call.

I believe God has been providing me with experiences in my life so I can share them with others who are traversing or have traversed these same roads. Having spent my toddler years in leg braces, teenage years in a biology lab, young adulthood as a medical secretary at Duke University Medical Center, and later as an assistant for an oxygen company, I have been living to learn and learning to live within the medical community, as well as through life's medical mayhem. As an adult, I became my mother's caregiver. By the time my husband survived not one but two rounds of cancer, I had become even more adept at navigating the medical arena.

But it wasn't until my own diagnosis of breast cancer in 2003, a follow-up hysterectomy the same year, and bypass surgery for coronary artery disease that I began applying Bible verses to difficult moments I was experiencing. I began to see my medical challenges as a way of growth. Daily devotions and Bible readings became a way to keep my life in perspective. Using humor to cushion the pain and God's Word in my heart and mind for strength, I have been able to maintain clarity and perseverance. As I shared these moments with others, I found that they were inspired to persevere as well.

At that point, I realized I finally had something to write about! I saw that what I did to cope and my perspective on medical issues just might help others navigate their medical issues on their way to eternity. American watercolor artist Bev Doolittle said it best: "I think that to find meanings, you have to look at things from different directions."

Through these short stories and their powerful messages, it is my hope that you will laugh, cry, learn about the health industry, and apply Bible verses to your life. These devotionals, for those who have undergone or are undergoing medical issues—whether your own or those of a loved one—will inspire you. I offer Bible verses for solace and comfort. It is my hope that this faith-centered book will provide the much-needed reminder that with God, all things are possible. In today's medical industry–and it is an industry–consumers must be equipped with all the armor they can possess. *Surviving Medical Mayhem* arms you with the knowledge you need to transform medical mayhem into confidence and serenity.

Disclaimer: This is not your average book of devotionals. I treat touchy subjects with grace and honesty. If you are looking for warm and fuzzy, smoothed-over events, or an escape from reality, this is not for you. It is real. It is blunt. And it is personal. But isn't life just that—blunt and personal, sometimes making you squirm? This book is written so that when you feel like you want to squirm, you have coping mechanisms to help you stand your ground and deal with those moments. It is my greatest desire and hope that you find help, hope, and humor as you read *Surviving Medical Mayhem*.

Let's start moving from medical mayhem to surviving and thriving!

CHAPTER ONE

A Funny Thing Happened on the Way to Eternity: Body Changes

1-1. INTRO BODY IMAGE

For you created my inmost being; you knit me to-gether in my mother's womb. I praise you because I am fearfully and wonderfully made; your works are wonderful, I know that full well.

Psalm 139:13–15

Beauty is subjective yet standardized by our culture and society. Beauty is also personal. How we think of ourselves can influence our behaviors and lives as a whole. I am talking about self-image. If we believe we are not good at sports, we defeat ourselves before we have even tried. If we never try, then failure becomes a self-fulfilling prophecy. Our self-image can make us or destroy us.

I think about how God sees us. We have value in God's eyes even before we're able to do anything on our own. And God has a plan for our lives from the very beginning. He is the Creator of our bodies and souls. We know from the Bible that God created us in His likeness and that He loves us as His children. We are certainly made heavenly and wonderfully! If we believe this to be true, we should have but one image of ourselves: beautiful! We may not be beautiful by this world's standard, but we are beautiful in God's eyes. That is all that matters.

As we venture through our days and find ourselves lamenting about our

Our self-image can make us or destroy us

bodies and our image as compared with society's opinion, we must remind ourselves that in holding on to that poor self-image, we are setting boundaries (limits) for our individual accomplishments. God has plans for us that are so outside any limits we or this world can set. Who are we to limit God's desires for us?

Knowing this, we can change our behaviors and ourselves by changing the pictures we carry in our minds.

. . .

1-2. NO ONE KNOWS YOUR BODY BETTER THAN YOU —

EXCEPT YOUR MOTHER

So I say to you: Ask and it will be given to you: seek and you will find: knock and the door will be opened to you.

Luke 11:8

In 1955, a mother gave birth to her third child and felt that something was wrong with her infant's legs. They did not look like those of her other two children. This baby girl's feet seemed to turn inward. The mother voiced her concerns to the pediatrician. He brushed them off, saying, "Her feet will adjust as she begins to walk."

The mother waited a few more months and noticed that her little girl's feet continued to turn in on their sides. She went to another pediatrician, who told her she was worrying too much. Following her mother's instinct, she sought a third opinion. This doctor "confirmed" what the two previous doctors had said: "There's nothing wrong with your daughter's feet. Once she begins walking, they'll be just fine. Quit worrying so much." His tone and demeanor communicated that she was a neurotic mother.

In her desperate prayers at night, she prayed for guidance. A small voice spoke to her, telling her to continue searching for a doctor who would listen.

Over the next few months, the mother kept busy by packing up the house and preparing for a move to Brazil, where her husband was to begin a new job. The mother worried that she would be unable to find good health care for her family, especially her daughter, whom she still believed had something wrong with her legs and feet. When she landed in São Paulo, Brazil, and got her family situated in their new home, this determined mother set out to find a pediatrician. She found one and made an appointment for her daughter, who was now nine months old.

As soon as the physician began examining the baby's legs, he looked at the mother sharply and asked, "Did you not see that her legs and feet are turned inward?"

The mother began to cry. Not only were her worst fears validated, but her prayer had been answered by finding this doctor.

It seemed that the baby girl had been born with elongated tendons on the inside of her legs, thus causing her to walk on the inside of her ankles.

"We need to get this child into braces immediately and pray to God that we are not too late to turn this around," the physician said gravely.

The little girl was fitted with heavy metal braces and shoes that she would wear for three years, night and day. The shoes were connected to each other by a metal bar, thus preventing her from walking. Her mother carried her wherever they went.

At the end of three years, the doctor removed the braces. No longer would the toddler need them. The little girl's feet were straight, and she walked and ran like all little children did at that age.

More than fifty years later, not only does that girl walk straight, but she grew up performing ballet and playing dodgeball, Chinese jump rope, basketball, volleyball, and racquetball. She also roller-skated and bicycled with her friends. She has physically been able to do anything and everything she wanted to do, without limitations.

That mother was my mother, and I was that little girl. If my father had not been transferred to Brazil and my mother had not continued to pursue what she knew was a health problem, I might never have walked—or if so, not comfortably. I might always have had a handicap of walking on the inside of my feet.

P.S.: I love buying shoes!

Surviving and Thriving

Nobody knows your body better than you, except maybe your mother. Seek God's help and wise counsel, and listen to the Holy Spirit. Then go with your heart. If you feel something is wrong, find a doctor who will listen to what you know: your body.

Prayer

Thank You, Father, for mothers who know their children, seek God's help, listen to the Holy Spirit, and follow their instincts in caring for them. And thank You for guiding us through troubled waters to safe passages.

• • •

1-3. AGE NOT BY NUMBER BUT BY LINGERIE

She is clothed with strength and dignity; she can laugh at the days to come.

Proverbs 31:25

Your beauty should not come from outward adornment, such as elaborate hairstyles and the wearing of gold jewelry or fine clothes. Rather, it should be that your inner self, the unfading beauty of a gentle and quiet spirit, which is of great worth in God's sight.

1 Peter 3:3-4

Our society bases age on a number, but I have learned that my age is not determined by turning fifty, sixty, seventy, or eighty…but by my lingerie.

As I grew out of diapers, I looked forward to wearing cute little Carter cotton underwear with unicorns and hearts. And let's not forget the briefs with the days of the week on them.

When I was a young adult, silky, tiny bikini underwear was a wardrobe must. It went along with the half bras that gave you cleavage that would make Mount Rushmore blush. Along with the long, flowing nightgowns and sweet baby-doll nighties, they made me feel like the beautiful young woman I was. Who isn't at age twenty to twenty-five?

As I matured into womanhood and matrimony, the doctor suggested cotton briefs to help prevent the infections that seemed to plague me. So I grudgingly made the switch for health's sake.

A hysterectomy, a lumpectomy, and a few persistent breast rashes at the radiation site led the doctors to prescribe white cotton bras, too! I hadn't worn cotton bras since I wore Carter panties and a training bra.

I have come full circle. Now the aging process is almost complete. I am just waiting until I am incontinent and the doctor prescribes Depends.

Surviving and Thriving

It's not the number that defines us, but how we wear it.

Prayer

Father God, it is not what is on the outside that matters to You but what is inside. I will see myself not as society sees beauty but as You do.

. . .

1-4. WHO'S IN BETTER SHAPE — THE CAR OR YOU?

You were bought at a price. Therefore, honor God with your body.

1 Corinthians 6:20

Ever since I was a young, married woman, I wanted a Volvo sedan. It was safe, solid, built to last, and beautiful. Brains, brawn, and beauty—who could want more? I would take good care of it. Thirty-two years later, I got my wish.

I love Vanessa Volvo. It's sleek, shiny, midnight black with gold speckles of color. Years ago, my brother told me, "If you take good care of a car, it will take good care of you." So I would clean it inside and out, buff it, wax it, and even clean the engine. I made sure to use the best gas and oil and regularly had the routine maintenance done.

Why don't we maintain our bodies at least as well as our cars?

Why is it that we will spend thousands of dollars getting the car we want and maintaining it, but we don't think twice about putting a Double Quarter Pounder with Cheese, super-sized fries, and a chocolate milkshake into our magnificently made bodies? Are our bodies not at least as important, if not more, than our cars? Why don't we maintain our bodies at least as well as our cars?

I have spent many a Christmas holiday season abusing my body by ingesting all kinds of preservative-laden, processed, and rich foods. I imagine the collection of food in my belly looking like a garbage dump. Chocolate (any type), sodas, chips, cookies, processed cheese spreads, candy, fast food, and alcohol are just a few of the foods I consume. To top off this abuse, I do very little in the way of exercise, except for grabbing more food off buffet tables. I am a glutton.

Throw in the stress of decorating the house, putting up the Christmas lights on the outside (they never work, no matter how carefully I stored them away the year before), shopping for just the right gifts, attending all the special events, baking twenty different kinds of cookies, and cooking the traditional holiday foods, and you have enough pressure to blow the top off Mount Vesuvius.

Before the holiday celebrations were over, I would begin to feel the effects of this disregard for my body. I would have the energy and enthusiasm of a tortoise. The thought of putting all that Christmas décor away made me cry out in utter despair.

Am I not worth at least as much energy and care as I give to Vanessa Volvo?

Why don't we take care of our bodies as well as we take care of our cars? Certainly it's much more advantageous. The life span of our bodies far outweighs the life span of any car—although the way I am taking care of this body, my Volvo will certainly outlast me.

Surviving and Thriving

We should take care of our own bodies as well as we take care of our cars. Think of all we could accomplish with this level of attention. Genetics still plays a role, but its negative effects may be deterred and its positive effects enhanced by the proper care and feeding of our bodies.

Prayer

Father God, my body is Your temple. You created this amazing body so I may follow in Your ways. I will nourish my body so I may be a wonderful example of Your love.

. . .

1-5. LOST AND FOUND

*He heals the brokenhearted and
binds up their wounds.*

Psalm 147:3

One morning, the phone rang. I picked it up and heard, "I lost my nipple."

No "Good morning." No "Hello."

It was my mother. She had just completed a series of operations that had reconstructed her breasts following a radical mastectomy. She now sported the breasts of a supermodel. Mine, at thirty-three, were sagging like weeping willow trees, where kids, monkeys, Tarzan, and Jane had hung on them. Hers were so perky I expected them to salute. There should be a law against mothers looking better than their daughters.

"Did you hear me?" my mother asked, bringing me back to the matter at hand...or at breast.

"What do you mean, you 'lost your nipple'?" I asked incredulously. "It's not like you can leave it somewhere."

"It's gone, I tell you. It just fell off."

"How?" I asked, still not quite believing it. Can nipples just fall off?

"Well, I was taking my bath this morning and washing up, and the next thing I know, it's sort of floating in the bathtub."

"Wow." I wasn't sure how else to respond.

"Yup, just floating around," my mom said as easily as "I am just floating in the Jacuzzi."

"So, what did you do?"

"I flushed it down the toilet."

"You did *what*!? Shouldn't we get it, pack it in ice and bring it back to the surgeon and maybe he can stitch it back on?"

"Well, it's only a nipple, for heaven's sake. I really don't need it. I still have my breasts! Just thought I should let someone know. Bye."

---

*Life isn't about being perfect.
It's about being in balance.*

I stared at the receiver before hanging up. Then I realized life isn't about being perfect. It's about being in balance. It isn't about being young but about being whole. It isn't about feeling sorry for yourself; it's about being able to move on in life. My mother felt that she could finally put her experience with cancer behind her. And she had two new breasts to help her do it.

Surviving and Thriving

Nothing in life is perfect. Find joy in all things, however small or seemingly insignificant.

Prayer

Father, God, help me remember where I have been and where I am today. Let me see the good that remains, even when something bad is happening. Thank You, Father, for giving me this second sight.

.   .   .

1-6. VANITY WILL GET YOU NOTHING,

EXCEPT MAYBE A TOILET TOUPEE

And why do you worry about clothes?
See how the flowers of the field grow.
They do not labor or spin.

Matthew 6:28

My mother had cancer and underwent chemotherapy, which caused her to lose her hair. Because she had always hated her hair (too frizzy, too thin, and too red), we told her that God was giving her a second chance and that when it grew back in, it would be thick, straight, and beautiful.

Mom and I went in search of the perfect wig. If there was a wig store within a one-hundred-mile radius, we were there! After more than four weeks of constant shopping, she settled on a $500 wig. It was made of human hair and had a cap-like netting to help keep Mom's head cool. It was straight, thick, and a beautiful shade of auburn.

One morning, Mom used her walker to get into the bathroom. She prepared to put on her new wig by placing a stocking cap over her very bald and smooth head. She put on the wig and adjusted it. She became frustrated because she felt that the hairs were not lying straight, and she asked if I would fix it. I looked at the wig—a pageboy cut with bangs—and not a hair seemed out of place. I told her so.

"Can't you see that the side and back just don't seem to lie right? Here, you take the pick and fix it," Mom said. Rather than argue, I thought it easier to take the pick and go through the motions of combing her wig straight.

Unfortunately, the pick caught the wig's netting just right, and the wig flew off my mother's smooth head, and the stocking cap stayed in place. The two of us watched in horror as the wig flew through the air, seemingly in slow motion, heading right for the toilet bowl. With both hands on her walker, my mother kept exclaiming, "Oh my! Oh my!"

All the while, I kept thinking, "Where are we going to get the money to replace this five-hundred-dollar rat...I mean wig?" Mom was between me and the bowl, and there was nothing we could do but watch as the wig hit the toilet seat, teetered for a moment, and then fell...onto the tile floor! We looked into the mirror at each other and burst out laughing.

Surviving and Thriving

It's what is on the inside that makes us beautiful on the outside.

Prayer

Abba, Father, our hearts and souls need care, for they are what make us beautiful! When our outer appearance becomes a source of strife, may we recall that we are all beautiful in Your sight. Physical beauty may be temporary, but the beauty within us will never die. Amen.

. . .

1-7. WHERE DO YOU RESIDE:

PENTHOUSE SUITE OR FIRST-FLOOR FLAT?

The L<small>ORD</small> *does not look at the things man looks at. People look at the outward appearance, but the* L<small>ORD</small> *looks at the heart.*

1 Samuel 16:7

When I was diagnosed with breast cancer, I had three options: (1) remove both breasts and use the fat from my belly to create new small breasts, (2) remove both breasts and replace them with implants, or (3) have a lumpectomy.

The first two options would certainly remove the cancer and my breasts, which were large and pendulous. They would be transformed into state-of-the-art, society-acceptable-and-appreciated, firm, well-formed breasts! The third option, a lumpectomy, would leave me with another scar. As I was considering the pros and cons, I decided that a consultation with a cosmetic surgeon was in order. I took my college-age daughter with me for support.

A young, beautiful, twenty-something nurse named Candy ushered us into an examining room and instructed me to disrobe. After the doctor came in, I explained my medical history and the purpose of my visit. He began to examine me by pushing my large, hanging breasts up to what seemed to me to be around my neck, or the penthouse suite (tenth floor). I suggested that I didn't want breasts that looked out of place with the rest of my forty-eight-year-old body. I pushed his hands to a lower position. He pushed them back up around my neck. I told him I wanted the breasts of a forty-something woman: full, firm, but with a bit of sag. I would be happy with breasts that lived on the eighth floor of my body rather than where they live , the third floor (my waist). They are racing each other to the first-floor flat.

He looked at his nurse, then at me, and I know he was thinking I was crazy. We discussed this a few minutes longer, with him pushing my breasts up and me pushing them down. My daughter was on the edge of her seat, poised to intervene in case I said something off color or shoved the doctor across the room—which had crossed my mind, I must confess.

Then I realized something.

I had grown into my breasts, and I was comfortable with them being just as they were. Society might define them as unattractive, but to me they had provided food for my daughter as an infant, created a soft pillow for my grandson to lie asleep in my arms, and offered a comforting place for my husband to rest his weary head and share the events of a long and difficult day. I had grown much attached (literally speaking) to my saggy breasts. They and the wrinkles on my face, and the rolls of fat in between, do not define me; they show where I have been and that I have survived. And I am okay with that.

My body and I reside where God and time placed them.

I ended the visit by thanking the doctor and his beautifully crafted nurse for their time. I took my low-swinging, sagging, third-floor breasts, as well as my full and slightly pear-shaped body, out the door with my back straight and my head held high. My body and I reside where God and time placed them. They are where they are meant to be.

I opted for the character-filled lumpectomy.

Surviving and Thriving

Where do you live in this world? Are you defined by your body? Do you let society dictate who you are by your body, or by your heart? Remember, you are more than the sum of your parts.

Prayer

I am on this Earth a short time, Father. You do not judge me by my body but by my soul. I want to keep my perspective when making decisions about my body so that the importance is on health, not on being eye candy for this world.

. . .

1-8. MY MANY SLEEPING PARTNERS

When pride comes, then comes disgrace, but with humility comes wisdom.

Proverbs 11:2

Ever since I turned fifty—the era of middle age—I have begun to have many sleeping partners. They pose no threat to my reputation or safety, and I am certain I will not catch anything from them. Let me introduce my sleeping partners to you:

- Chunky monkey—the knee wedge, which takes pressure off my back.

- Michelin tire wrap—the breast compression garment, which lessens the lymphedema in my breast due to a lumpectomy for breast cancer.

- The chastity bra—a sports bra, to house the compression garment that lessens the lymphedema in my breast.

- The giraffe collar—a neck collar that relieves the pressure in my neck when I sleep and helps prevent my fingers in my right hand from going numb.

- Snufflelupagus (remember the *Sesame Street* character?)—A CPAP machine, for my sleep apnea.

Each of these beauties came from the recommendation of a different physician—all to aid and return me to optimum health. None of my doctors realize just how long it takes me to get ready for bed at night. And I am not talking about applying creams and masks.

Let me share my nightly ritual with you. I prepare myself to retire by removing my glasses, washing my face, brushing my teeth, combing my hair, and performing my last basic bathroom visit before removing my day clothes and putting on what should be comfortable sleeping clothes. This sounds perfectly normal, right? Wait, it gets twisted.

Until recently, my next step was to put on a two-sizes-too-small sports bra (chastity bra) to house the compression garment (Michelin tire wrap). The tire wrap is a fully stuffed quilted piece that fits over the affected breast *inside* the two-sizes-too-small bra and wraps around to the back of my body. You have to be Houdini to get in and out of it, and I usually needed my husband's assistance to perform this trick. Recently I upgraded and now sport a zip-up Michelin tire (a compression garment that resembles a corset that closes with Velcro).

Okay, so once I have the Michelin tire wrap and the chastity bra on, I have to turn on the overhead fan because I am having a hot flash. *Whew!* Now I am ready for my nightgown. None of my nice nightgowns fit over the Michelin tire wrap with the chastity bra, so I settle for something easy, like an oversized nightshirt—very romantic.

Now I am ready for Snuffie. I place the strap and gear over my head and tweak the mask to fit "comfortably" (who are they kidding?) and adjust the hose leading from my mask to the machine that sits on my nightstand—

hence the name Snufflelupagus—so that it is out of my way. I then add the neck brace (giraffe collar) to complete the ensemble. The look is one of having been in a serious accident. I climb into bed and place the knee wedge (chunky monkey) between my legs. Now I am ready to have a wonderful night's sleep, right?

Wrong. Have you ever tried to sleep with all these partners? Every time I turn or change position, so do my partners. If I am lucky, I get a couple of hours of sleep at night. My friends wonder why I look so tired with being re-tired and no children living with us. I tell them it's just my sleeping partners keeping me up at night. And don't ask me to tell you what I have to do if the phone should ring or the cat throws up or one of the dogs is frantically signaling me that it needs to go out one last time. To make matters worse, by the time I complete my nighttime ritual, I often have to go to the bathroom.

I haven't had this much activity in bed since I woke up with fleas from sharing the bed with my dog. I asked my daughter if our grandson would be disturbed by my attire should he come into our room during the nights he is visiting. And then there is my husband's point of view of his lovely bride to consider. It's a wonder he still sleeps with me. I know he loves me and surely he understands, or soon will.

You see, my husband recently went to his internist because he is sleeping poorly. Seems he has a deviated septum, breathes through his mouth, and has just been prescribed his very own Snufflelupagus with a chin strap. Who knows, maybe I can get him to wear my chastity bra and Michelin tire wrap. I could sure use a break!

Surviving and Thriving

Father, although I am sleeping with chunky monkey and Snufflelupagus while stuffed in a too-tight chastity bra with a Michelin tire wrap jammed in it and a giraffe collar, I am grateful that those sleeping partners are there to help me.

Prayer

Help us to give thanks in all circumstances, even those that are difficult to appreciate. We do not need to be thankful *for* the difficult times, but help us to be thankful *in* the difficult times.

. . .

1-9. A PARALLEL UNIVERSE

He will renew your life and sustain you
in your old age.

Ruth 4:15

While visiting our grandson, Aiden, to celebrate his seventh birthday, I was struck by the similarities in our lives.

Aiden had just crossed the threshold from kindergarten to first grade. I had just turned sixty. We were both entering a new time in our lives.

In kindergarten, they introduce reading. First grade brings about major time and effort spent on reading full sentences–a requirement by the end of the school year. It was a monumental task for Aiden, who found words a challenge but had an aptitude for numbers (something I do not have). He needed a desk in his room because with first grade comes homework. Now that he was older, he had some maintenance that he needed to remember to do for himself rather than have his parents do or remind him to do–chores such as bathing, teeth brushing, making his bed, and feeding the dog and cat. He didn't mind doing them, and he tried hard to remember, but the chores cut into his playtime.

Likewise, I had entered a time in my life of many changes, and things were going on that really put a damper on my "playtime" as well. My body was wearing earlier than I imagined it would. My body obviously did not get the memo that sixty is the new fifty; it was acting as if it was eighty. The maintenance on this body had increased by at least 40 percent.

Although I no longer needed to shave my legs, renegade hairs grew in all the wrong places, requiring daily inspection and removal. That required magnifying mirrors and bifocal glasses, and I still missed some errant hairs. There were moisturizers for dry skin, hair thickeners and potions for thinning hair, age-defying products to cover up the wrinkles and age spots, and a plethora of other regimens that required instructions and a calendar to remind me to do them. And we won't discuss the vitamins and medicines that are prescribed to keep me going, glowing, and healthy.

Yes, it has really cut into my fun. Or has it?

You see, all this came to me at 2:00 a.m. while sitting in "the loo" of our hotel room at the Marriott on the eve of Aiden's birthday. I ended up spending more time than I had planned, mainly because my hips had deteriorated to a point where I needed to use a toilet that sits a bit higher. I could sit down on the toilet with ease, but getting up was difficult. Maybe it was the three-hour trip in the car or the four hours getting in and out of a car that same day looking at Orlando real estate, but my hips were clearly shouting, "Oh, no! We won't go!"

I was in a heck of a position, wasn't I? As I strategized how to lift myself up, I started to giggle. I could wake up my blissfully sleeping husband, but why should we both be sleepless in Orlando? I could lean back and just wait

---

*Change is inevitable whether
you are seven or sixty.*

---

until Thad woke up to answer his call of nature. However, with my luck, I would fall asleep and then slide off the toilet seat and onto the floor. Better not take the chance. I assessed my surroundings and considered my options. Grabbing onto the paper holder (praying it would hold) and the side of the tub, I rocked back and forth and launched myself into a standing position. Mission accomplished!

Life is a series of thresholds. Change is inevitable whether you are seven or sixty. Aiden and I were in parallel universes, each crossing a threshold. It required adjustment - a handicap accessible hotel room comes to mind followed closely by a hip replacement". Both of us would stretch and grow gracefully, and sometimes not so gracefully, accepting the new, the scary, and the exciting lives we have. And we would need to find the humor in the absurdity and the positions that we found ourselves in.

Surviving and Thriving

"There is a thin line that separates laughter and pain, comedy and tragedy, humor and hurt. If you can't make it better, you can laugh at it." –Erma Bombeck

Prayer

Omnipotent Father, when simple things in life become complicated, help me readily see the humor, not just the discomfort. May I find comfort in knowing that we are all on this earthly ride and will eventually arrive at the same place–the throne of Your glory!

. . .

1-10. REPURPOSING FOR A BEAUTIFUL AND PURPOSEFUL LIFE

Therefore, if anyone is in Christ, he is a new creation. The old has gone, the new has come.

2 Corinthians 5:17

Thad and I went looking for dining-room furniture. My brother and his wife have enjoyed many years of consignment and antique shopping and suggested that they take us to several of their favorite haunts. We spent two weekends going with them, and I am not sure what was more fun: looking for a find or watching them look for that something special to add to their home. We learned about the different eras of furniture and their "special-ness." We discovered a whole new world of beautiful treasures and some-thing about ourselves as well.

In a store called Deja New, surrounded by tables, chairs, sofas, lamps, and bric-a-brac, stood a tall and stately honey-colored wood curio cabinet with curved glass and clawed feet that had been built in the late 1800s. It had a shelf missing, some roughness in its wood, nicks and scuff marks around its edges, and years of dust and neglect. The light, although working, showed wiring that was worn and dangerous. Regardless, the curio cabinet spoke to us of long-ago family gatherings and memories that had been made and showcased in it. Despite its worn appearance, we fell in love with it and de-cided to bring it home.

My brother and sister-in-love gave me a Beginners' Wood Restoring 101 class. Using tack cloths, ultrafine steel wool, soft cloths, and Howard's refin-ishing polish, I began to wipe away the years of rough treatment and neglect. I went over the nicks and gouges until the wood was smooth and shone brightly. Although the cabinet still missed the one glass shelf, Thad replaced the light and its wiring.

God has been refinishing me through each of these events

As I worked on the cabinet, I began to see the analogy between this antique cabinet and me. Although I was made in God's image to be beautiful, life events and surgeries have marked me, scarred me, and changed me into what I am today. I am missing a few parts: an appendix; a cancerous lump; and an orchard of benign tumors, polyps, and fibroids. I no longer look shiny and new. And I have the scars to prove it. God has been refinishing me through each of these events (sometimes with steel wool a whole lot courser than extra-fine). When I am cleaned up, I still look older, and some of life's scars are evident.

But just like our new curio cabinet, I am repurposed. What I have lost in mobility, agility, and mental acuity, I have gained in prayer time, wisdom, maturity, and strength in faith. I have learned that it's not about my shiny finish but more about my content, my history, and my soul. The events in my past, both good and bad, have made me into something new. I am repurposed for a beautiful and purposeful life in Christ. After all, He uses crackpots–why not a worn, slightly scuffed, and roughed-up curio cabinet like me?

I stood back to admire "her" beauty. The cabinet was restored–not like it was originally–no, it would never be quite the same. In a way, it was better. Refined by age, and still showing some battle scars, its strength showed through. Renewed and repurposed, it gained a new sense of presence and a specialness that often characterizes things that are old. It was beautiful.

Surviving and Thriving

Like the old curio cabinet, we sport the scars of illnesses, surgeries, and life's habits, hurts, and hang-ups. Those we survive can make us more resilient, wiser, and stronger. In our own unique way, we are truly God's masterpieces.

Prayer

Merciful Father, help us see ourselves not as the world sees us, but as the beautiful mosaic works of art that you have created through living, loving, and life.

· · ·

1-11. IGNORE OR EXPLORE?

Place your trust in the Eternal; rely on Him completely; never depend upon your own ideas and inventions. Give Him the credit for everything you accomplish, and He will smooth out and straighten the road that lies ahead.

Proverbs 3:56 (The Voice)

Why was I more freaked out over having a biopsy of a blemish on my scalp than I was over my lumpectomy, or my coronary artery bypass?

It had been a few years since I had had a "body check" for skin lesions, and having found a spot on the back of my leg, I decided it was time. The doctor told me the spot was a blemish that often occurs as people age. More lumps and bumps in the natural course of getting old. Harrumph! However, the doctor asked, "How long have you had this bluish mark on the top of your head? We might want to biopsy this."

"I don't know," I responded, "but I will ask my hairstylist and get back to you."

My conversation with the hairstylist resulted in making an appointment with the dermatologist to have the "bluish blemish" biopsied. And that is when my mind went into overdrive. Would they shave my scalp or put a bandage on my head that I would later have to yank off, taking with it the few hairs I have left on my thinning scalp? And how would I look going to the women's retreat the next day, sporting a bald spot or a bandage? Would I be left with a naked spot that would require imported hair to cover up because at my age, nothing seems to come back except my weight?

I thought about the other skin biopsies I had had over the years and how the results had been negative. This could be no different. I don't need a biopsy, right? But then, I never wear a hat when I am out in the sun because it is either uncomfortable, hot, or blows away in the wind unless I have it anchored like a ship to a dock. Maybe I should have it biopsied. *But I don't want to have it biopsied!*

Could it be that I was so vain that losing a little bit of hair would stop me from doing what was healthy? Could I ignore this, hope it disappeared, and do so without worry? And if it really was melanoma—what then?

Was I vain enough to ignore it or wise enough to grab onto my faith and deal with it?

Taking my obsessive worry and fear to the Lord, I realized I had a choice in this matter, and that was why it was difficult. With my lumpectomy and coronary artery bypass, I had no such choice. Those courses of action were definitive and required. This simple procedure was an elective choice—well, sort of. It was a decision I needed to make, one in which wisdom, or the lack thereof, would determine the future of my health.

The day of the biopsy came. I lifted up prayers to God in the car just before going into the doctor's office. I made the best decision I could make and then put my trust in God for the outcome. That being said, it didn't stop me from pouring out all my concerns and sounding like a Wendy Whiner

Perfect peace is not dependent on circumstances

or Vanessa, the Aging and Vain Vamp. But the nurse and the doctor were patient and kind. Nothing was shaved, and nothing was bandaged. A shot to numb my head, a small hole punch to sample the skin, a few stitches, and a dab of antibiotic ointment, and I was out the door with nothing more than a headache and sticky, disheveled hair.

I had to wait a few days for the report. Regardless of the results, I knew that as long as I made my decisions with God in the equation, I could leave the outcome to the Father, too.

Surviving and Thriving

Making choices can be difficult when we would rather put our heads in the sand than stare straight into the sun. But make them anyway. Your life may depend on it.

Prayer

Heavenly Father, perfect peace is not dependent on circumstances. Rather, it comes from a steadfast, trusting heart focused on You. Help me make decisions despite my fear and to know that courage is merely fear that has said its prayers.

. . .

1-12. HUMOR THERAPY

A joyful heart is good medicine, but a broken
spirit dries up the bones.

Proverbs 17:22 (NASB)

Two weeks after Thad's shoulder surgery, I was beginning to wear down. How was I going to maintain stamina, not to mention the right attitude? Unless he had some miraculous healing, there would be four more weeks of bathing the two of us, dressing the two of us, and feeding the two of us. If it weren't for the humor that peppers our days, that season of our lives might have been unbearable.

Immediately after surgery, I found Thad hooked up to an electrical cooling system that transported cold water from a container filled with ice and water to a blue cold pack he wore on his shoulder. Two long hoses went from the container and attached to two shorter hoses that were on his blue shoulder pack. The two shorter hoses looked like New Age cow udders hanging off his right arm. On top of the cooling system was a black shoulder sling, and on his right arm and shoulder was a bolster. A smaller bolster, with the aid of Velcro, could be attached anywhere. A black exercise ball attached by Velcro to the top of his arm completed his ensemble. We had spent a lot of time trying to determine exactly who he reminded us of. The possibilities were endless: Inspector Gadget (if you remember the cartoon series), a retired transformer, a Darth Vader wannabe, or a Star Trek Borg.

We had to learn how to hook up the entire apparatus because he was to use this for six weeks. The cooling system was easy once we remembered which direction the udders had to go. The sling was a bit tricky; it had clips and straps, not all of which were used or needed. Taking it off was easy. But remembering what clipped into what could be problematic at the end of a long day when we were both tired. Thad and I often quipped that, at our age, it took the two of us to make one brain. It must have been funny watching the one-armed, retired transformer and a frazzled, brain-drained, menopausal woman accomplish this feat.

Then there was the exercise ball. One of the first things Thad said to me when he came out of the operating room was, "Look, Honey, I got my ball back!" It was then I knew that he would be fine. You see, Thad had testicular cancer, not once but twice. People often ask him if he is concerned that his cancer will return. He always replies, "No, I am out of balls!"

This little ball provided us with many moments of laughter. I told him that if he didn't do everything Nurse Loretta said, I would take it away from him.

On one of his first nights home from the hospital, our good friend, Jan, brought us dinner. What a blessing. We asked her to join us. As she and I were serving the fettuccini and meatballs, we both simultaneously realized Thad might not be able to eat it because his right arm and hand were in the sling. She was mortified and apologetic for causing a problem rather than helping. I figured it could be a scene from *Dirty Rotten Scoundrels*, where Steve Martin acts like he is Michael Cain's brother, who is mentally challenged. In the movie, he acts brain-addled when eating, nearly poking his eyes out with the fork. I told Jan not to worry, and I offered to feed Thad.

But Thad was nonplussed. He picked up the fork with his left hand and began to twirl the fettuccini like a true Italian. Not a drop of sauce went flying, and not a bit of pasta flung around his plate. And he managed to get it into his mouth. Well, that was like waving a red flag and challenging two bulls. Jan and I both picked up our forks with our left hands and proceeded to send fettuccini and sauce all over the table. Who needed to feed whom here?

After two weeks, it was hard to imagine another four with the sling and bolster. When it was over, we had a solemn service as we burned it over a trash can. But not before we had lots of laughter in between.

Surviving and Thriving

What a wonderful, unexpected joy to laugh spontaneously at the little things that make an awkward or difficult moment easier. If we look at only the difficulty in our lives, then that is all we see. But if in the midst of those difficult moments we can find a bit of humor, a slice of sweetness, or a cup of love, then life is endurable, doable, and even surmountable.

Prayer

Father, life can be difficult. But You have provided us with the ability to laugh. I ask that You help us find the humor in the adversity in our lives. For it is in the humor that we can help ourselves and forge through the pain.

· · ·

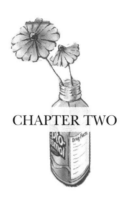

CHAPTER TWO

I Would've Taken Better Care of Myself Had I Known What Would Happen: Taking Care of Ourselves

2-1. INTRO: WE ARE WORTHY OF HIS CARE

*So don't be afraid, you are worth
more than many sparrows.*

Matthew 10:31

If love directs and guides us to care for others, then can't love be the guide for caring for ourselves? The caveat is that caring for ourselves is measurable by how much we truly love and respect ourselves. And therein lies the rub, my friends. Many of us have messages running through our thoughts, like a CD stuck on replay–messages we were told, taught, believed, and now tell ourselves: "You are not good enough, you will never be successful, you do not measure up, and you are not worthy."

I spent most of my life believing these lies. I took them all in and truly felt unworthy. Sometimes I still fight the bad self-talk. I am worthy of caring for others but am unworthy of caring for myself or being cared for. Yet I desperately desire and need to care for myself.

The Bible tells us that God created us in His own likeness and that He loves us, no matter what wrongs we have committed in action, thought, and deed. He even uses those ills for good! And if He uses those poor choices, can you imagine what He would do with a healthy body, mind, and soul? Maybe we feel empowered when we show we are caring for others but find no pleasure in caring for ourselves.

Caring for yourself is caring for God's temple

However, I suggest that caring for yourself is caring for God's temple, and caring for God's temple builds strong followers who, in turn, can truly make a difference in the world.

This chapter explores the various ways you can care for yourself. Taking time to be with God, knowing your family history, learning how your body works, listening to your body, and recognizing its needs will help you align yourself with the temple that God created for you and you alone–your body.

. . .

2-2. BODY BY GOD, DISCOVERY BY CHILD

Let the wise hear and increase in learning, and the one who understands obtain guidance.

Proverbs 1:5 (ESV)

It's important to learn everything you can about your body. Mark Van Doren, who was an English professor at Columbia University for forty years, said it well: "Any piece of knowledge I acquire today has a value at this moment exactly proportioned to my skill to deal with it. Tomorrow, when I know more, I recall that piece of knowledge and use it better."

From the moment we are born and our eyes begin to focus, we are gaining knowledge by exploring the world around us. We explore our hands and feet as they cross into our path of vision. We discover our belly buttons and touch every part of them, learning every fold and crevice. As toddlers, we continue exploring the world not only around us but within us. This marvelous time of discovery continues until we become complacent and develop a laissez-faire attitude about our bodies. It's as if we get bored, no longer care, or have no time for them. We want them to run on their own. How our bodies run depends largely on how we have learned to keep them clean, nourished, and maintained.

Knowledge is empowering

Some of us would prefer that our primary physicians told us what to do and did not explain the details or reasons. Others partner with their primary physicians, learning and never ceasing to explore the infinite intricacies of the human body. I believe we should always remain aware of our bodies because they are constantly providing us feedback, ever-changing in their nature, and are always fascinating. Knowledge is empowering.

When we don't explore, learn, investigate, and care for our bodies, we often experience pain, fear, and frustration. Two stories illustrate this point.

As my mom, Gloria, approached her ninth birthday, her mother instructed the nanny to sleep in Mom's room. The nanny didn't know why, and she didn't ask. Information in the household was on a need-to-know basis, and the children were rarely in the position of needing to know. One night, my mother woke up and felt kind of "icky." She went to the bathroom and discovered that her PJ bottoms were covered in blood. She sat there for a moment, wondering when she could have been shot. Why did she not hear the gun? She felt sort of achy, but surely she would feel more pain if she had been shot. Was she dying? As she was contemplating this, the nanny came in, helped clean her, and provided the necessary supplies. She assured her that her mother would explain everything in the morning.

The dawn of the day did bring explanation from her mother that she was a woman now and that every month she would get this "showing." My grandmother made it a point to tell my mom not to share this information with anyone, especially her little sister. It was serious, personal, and private. Being the dutiful daughter, my mother kept it to herself—until her sister got wind of something secret.

Her younger sister, my aunt, knew that these cotton things (feminine hygiene pads) came out of my mother's closet every so often, but when she asked about them, my mother told her to mind her own business. Well, that was like sounding the horn for battle. Over the course of the next few months, whenever my aunt would find these cotton things, she would tie them to the handlebars of her bicycle and run around the neighborhood yelling, "Gloria's pads for sale! Get Gloria's pads today!" Sometimes when my mother had friends over, my aunt would come into the room, swinging them like a flapper girl swinging her beads or boa. True story! Talk about pain in ignorance.

The second story is also about Mom. My mother was never told about the facts of life (why are you not surprised?), yet at age seventeen, she met and married my father. Can you imagine how surprised both my mother and father were on their wedding night? My father knew that his bride was a virgin, but he thought she knew the basic itinerary for the honeymoon. To my mother, the gentleman had turned from Dr. Jekyll to Mr. Hyde!

Suffice it to say that my father was an extremely patient husband and slowly taught my mother about the love shared between a man and a woman. My mother related to me how angry she was at her parents for not sharing this knowledge that would have made her life less stressful and would have helped her enjoy her wedding night. But what could have ended a marriage before it had begun turned into twenty-five shared years together.

Because of those two events in her life, my mother made sure I was well prepared and understood my body, its purpose, and its function. I thank God for the wisdom my mother had to learn the hard way.

Surviving and Thriving

Living with your body is so much easier when you seek to know everything you possibly can about it.

Prayer

Lord, help me to seek and explore this wonderful body and world You created and to remember that wisdom can grow from all experiences. I will seek, explore, learn, and grow in this body You created for me. Like a child, I will never cease to appreciate my body. Thank You for my body.

. . .

2-3. CIVIL WAR

How good and pleasant it is when God's people live together in unity!

Psalm 133:1

Brain. Hey, collective body, let's go out and wash the car.

Body. That's great! Good exercise for us.

So the brain and the body work together, and soon the car looks great.

Brain. While I am out here, I could do some weeding. We'll clear the weeds from under this weeping hibiscus.

Body. Fair enough. Bending exercises are good for me.

Time goes by; the brain keeps adding "exercises" for the body to do. The body is getting tired.

Body. Wow! Listen, you didn't provide me with enough water and food for all this activity.

The body begins to come undone.

Back. Yeah, and I'm getting tired of holding up the top part of the body throughout all of this.

Shoulders. Well, it's no picnic here, you know.

Head. I feel like I am going to explode.

Throat. I, for one, am dry and parched…but not for long. Stomach is heaving up some stuff, and it's really gross.

Stomach. It's not my fault. I'm feeling a little queasy. I think that inner-ear thing is going on again.

Ears/Eyes. Hey, I am not to blame here. What do you expect? I have to look through these bifocals, and she keeps moving up and down, over this way, then that way. I don't feel so well myself.

Brain. Okay, just hold it together, guys. I just really want to get the rest of the front beds weeded, and then we will stop.

So the body bucks up under the pressure. But when the brain starts thinking about pulling out the pruning shears, all the body parts groan and moan in unison.

Body. Hey, Brain, lighten up. We're all sick. This is more than you told us you were going to do.

Brain. Yeah, I know, but with the weeding done, I see I need to prune.

Body. Prune? You want to see pruning? We'll show you pruning!

With that, a complete rebellion takes place, and the brain realizes he has lost control. He gives up, but the body can barely move. Sweat is pouring, hands and knees are shaking, heartbeat is accelerating. The body is cold and clammy. The body is in trouble.

Brain. Hey, guys! What's going on? What happened?

Body. Listen, we told you to stop after the weeds were pulled out from under the hibiscus. But no, you had stuff to do. We told you to stop after the front beds were weeded. Did you listen? We begged you to quit before you started pruning. But *noooo!* You think we can just go on forever. You didn't give us enough fluids—last night's wine didn't count or help—and coffee and toast aren't enough breakfast for this kind of work. Just because you think doesn't mean you're the boss!

It took the body what little it had left to get it into that dull brain just what was happening.

Brain. *Sheepish.* Okay, okay.

The brain listens to the body and goes into the house. Now the brain is focused on all the parts of the body, for it is in bad shape. Advil, water, a banana, more water, and a two-hour rest period are necessary before the body is restored to usefulness. The brain has learned a lesson, at least until the next time it thinks it is superior to the rest of the body.

Surviving and Thriving

It takes both the body and the brain to work in concert to maintain what God has created: a masterpiece.

Prayer

Thank You, God, for giving us our amazing bodies with all their different parts, each an integral part of the whole. We must care for each part equally so that the whole may be able to do the work for which You created us.

．　．　．

2-4. I CAN DO IT ALL BY MYSELF

We have different gifts, according to the grace given us. If a man's gift is prophesying, let him use it in proportion to his faith. If it is serving, let him serve; if it is teaching, let him teach; if it is encouraging, let him encourage; if it is contributing to the needs of others, let him give generously; if it is leadership, let him govern diligently; if it is showing mercy, let him do it cheerfully.

Romans 12:6–8

I was four days out from my coronary artery bypass and still in the hospital, but all IVs, catheters, and tubes had been removed. I woke up one night feeling like I was in a coal furnace.

I decided to get out of bed and lower the air conditioning in my hospital room. Although I was on the healing road, getting in and out of bed was a long, protracted ordeal. First, I would remove all pillows I used to hug against my chest and support my back. I would hook my legs on the side of the bed and use them to pull me up enough to get on my elbow. Then I would use my stomach muscles (the ones that had been cut into twice in prior operations, i.e., they were nonexistent) to sit up on the side of the bed and wait until I could catch my breath. From there, it was easy street!

I tottered to the thermostat, which was just outside the door to my hospital room, when I realized I needed my glasses to see the settings. I hobbled back into my room, put on my glasses, shuffled back to the doorway, and adjusted the thermostat to make it cooler in the room. Then I went back to sit on the bed and reversed the painstaking process until I was in a supine position.

Whew! I was tired. As I lay there, I realized I still had my glasses on. I removed them and placed them beside me in bed. No, that would not do. I could roll on them and bend them, or worse. I needed to put them on the nightstand, but I was lying with my back to the stand. I reached behind me to place them on the stand. They promptly fell onto the floor. I was so tired and out of breath by that point, I considered leaving them on the floor until I got up later in the night.

But I knew the nurses would be in to check my blood pressure, and the vampires–I mean lab techs–would be in to get their quota of blood from me. They could step on my glasses, which would end up crunched and broken. I would be blind as a bat without radar.

I began the laborious process of getting up again when I realized I couldn't! All I could do was press the call button for the nurse and wait for help. Within minutes, a nurse was there and picked up my glasses, helped me get settled, and scolded me for not calling her sooner.

After I was situated, I began thinking about learning what you can and

---

At certain times, we must ask for help

---

cannot do and realizing that at certain times, we must ask for help. I was reminded of how upset I was when a friend of mine was slowly becoming caged by multiple sclerosis and would not accept help from family or friends. My glasses incident showed me that I was being just like my dear friend. I needed to give my body time to heal. My stubbornness and my pride were inhibiting that process.

Surviving and Thriving

Knowing when to call in the reserves is important for our emotional, physical, and spiritual well-being. It allows us to receive the help we need and lighten our load so that we may heal. It allows givers the opportunity to share their gift of caregiving. In every way, both parties are given gifts.

Prayer

Father God, thank You for giving each of us gifts and for the opportunities to share our gifts during different seasons of our lives. Sometimes we are the givers, and sometimes we are the receivers. In all times, help us to listen to our bodies' needs and hear Your desires for us through words, Scripture, and those around us. When we think we are doing it all by ourselves, help us remember that it is only by Your grace that we do so.

. . .

2-5. HIPPO IN A BUSINESS SUIT

*Trust in the Lord with all your heart and
lean not on your own understanding.
In all ways, acknowledge Him and He will
lead your paths straight.*

Proverbs 3:5–6

My husband, Thad, had testicular cancer not once but twice—the right testicle at age thirty-two and the left testicle at age forty-seven. Thad tells everyone that there will be no recurrence; after all, he's out of supplies.

His first surgery was followed by eight weeks of radiation therapy. When he was diagnosed the second time, Thad thought that because they couldn't do radiation again, chemotherapy was in his future. As a pharmaceutical rep having sold cancer drugs, he knew just enough to be dangerous. He figured the chemo would make him sick. He decided he might as well eat himself through the holidays. He began with the diagnosis in November and didn't stop eating until a consult visit on December 31 at Indiana University Medical Center, where some of the leading testicular cancer research was being conducted.

During that appointment, Thad learned that, because of his relatively young age, they did not recommend chemotherapy. Rather, they would closely monitor him for the following five years with blood tests, CT scans, X-rays, and so on. They explained that patients his age who received prophylactic chemotherapy later experienced side effects such as heart failure. At that moment, he realized he might have a problem. He knew he had eaten quite a bit of food and packed on a few pounds. He had been living in pull-on shorts and sweat suits since his surgery, so he didn't realize the extent of it.

Two days after his consult, he found out just how many pounds he had gained. Thad was preparing to return to work and would be attending a business meeting out of town. I was washing all his clothes, and he was picking out his business suits for the trip. As I entered our bedroom with a stack of freshly cleaned and folded clothes, I heard what could only be described as cacophony followed by some very strong exclamations. It seemed to be coming from our clothes closet. I imagined that the shelf had come down with the weight of the clothes hanging from it.

Not so, Sherlock! What I saw next was so funny that I had to sit down on our hope chest for fear that I would drop the pile of clothes and soil my underwear.

Thad came out of the closet wearing a pair of suit pants that looked like they were at least three sizes too small. The constriction pushed the fat up above his waist and made his chest area look like that of a hippopotamus… or maybe the Michelin Man.

His face was beet red. He huffed and puffed and said, "If I had known I wasn't going to have chemo, I wouldn't have eaten so much!"

Of course, my laughter didn't help calm him, but it sure helped me release eight weeks of stored-up worry. It took a trip to Men's Wearhouse and the loss of fifteen pounds before Thad was able to join me in laughing about the time he looked like a hippo in a business suit.

Surviving and Thriving

Never assume and consume, for the waist will make haste to waste.

Prayer

Our Father, only You know what our future holds. No matter what that future is, You are with us. Thank You, Father, for Your understanding and for loving us in spite of our temptations to assume the course of our future.

. . .

2-6. FOR CRYING OUT LOUD

The Lord's favor is for a lifetime.
Weeping may linger for the night, but joy
comes with the morning.

Psalm 30:5 (GWT)

There have been times in my life when I felt overwhelmed by so many medical issues (mine, my mother's, and my husband's) that I just wanted to cry. However, I would hold it in, whether it was because I was putting on a good front, trying to avoid upsetting anyone, or worrying that others would think less of me if I broke down. So I did what every good Type A personality does: I scheduled my cries. Yup, you read it correctly. I would wait until I knew I was going to be alone. Then and only then would I let my guard down and just sob. I felt like a crazy loon singing at sunset! But a strange thing always happened following my cries even though the problems were still there, I felt better.

There is validity to the phrase "a good cry." Research has shown that although you end up with red and swollen eyes, shed tears are a panacea for distress and can lead to a healthy mind and body. Tears help keep foreign matter from one's eyes, keep the eye membrane hydrated, and contain lysozyme, which help kill bacteria.[1]

Research from Dr. William Frey found that tears caused by grief or stress contain toxins and stress hormones that exit the body through tears; however, tears shed because of peeling onions or getting a speck of dirt in your

---

1. Lizette Borelli, "Cry It Out: Six Surprising Health Benefits of Shedding a Few Tears," Medical Daily, May 19, 2015, http://www.medicaldaily.com/cry-it-out-6-surprising-health-benefits-shedding-few-tears-333952.

eye do not release those same toxins or hormones.[2] So fighting back tears instead of having a good cry can keep those nasty toxins and hormones inside. Yuk!

Like exercise, crying can also reduce stress by releasing endorphins and prolactin and helps fight diseases caused by stress, such as high blood pres-

---

Crying can also reduce stress

---

sure. It will improve your mood and make you feel more relaxed. While crying, your body goes through a series of chemical changes that actually mellow you and can even help you sleep better.

After I have one of my scheduled cries, I always feel a sense of relief. Crying certainly hasn't solved my problems, but my ability to deal with them is enhanced. So whether you schedule a cry or just need to cry on the spot, for crying out loud, do so!

Surviving and Thriving

Although our society has taught us to hold our emotions inside and never let anyone see us cry, scientific proof shows that crying is beneficial. Don't be afraid to cry out loud. Your health depends on it.

Prayer

Creator of heaven and Earth and all living creatures, how amazing are the bodies You created for us. Thank You for creating such a system that purifies, cleanses, and restores us to the beings You created us to be.

. . .

---

2. "The Stress-Reducing Benefits of Crying," StressSilence, June 26, 2013, http://www.silencestress.com/crying-relieves-stress/.

2-7. THE PB&J SANDWICH

And we know that in all things God works for the good of those who love him, who have been called according to His purpose.

Romans 8:26 (NIV)

While walking the dogs one day, I ran into a neighbor who had recently moved her mother into her home to live with her. I asked her how she was doing. Between home-schooling her ten-year-old and caring for her mom, who was beginning to decline physically, a mixture of emotions, negative thoughts, and mental and physical exhaustion came forth like hot lava pouring onto the sidewalk.

In those few moments, I found myself transported back twenty-five years, when I found myself in a similar position in my life. This position even has a name.

Called the "Sandwich Generation," it is defined as "a generation of people, typically in their thirties or forties, responsible for bringing up their own children while caring for their aging parents." At the time, I did not know my situation had a name, but I sure could feel it. I felt pressed and perplexed, inept and inferior, and in demand yet invisible–all at the same time.

I was barely thirty, and my daughter Francesca was three. My mother

---

I felt pressed and perplexed

---

was fifty-eight when she had breast reconstruction following a radical mastectomy for cancer. In a series of three surgeries, I had just brought her home from the second surgery, during which they had removed the muscle from her back and placed it in her chest wall. She was in extreme pain, so I brought her to my home to convalesce for a day or two.

That evening, my three-year-old daughter developed a fever, chills, and malaise. I was running between the guest room and my daughter's room until, exhausted, I moved them both into the bed my husband and I shared. I knew I was "sandwiched" when my mother was moaning in excruciating pain and my daughter began talking incoherently from the fever. I quickly ran a tepid bath and submerged Francesca's body into it to break her 104-degree temperature. It was not an easy task because she was crying, screaming, and begging me to stop as she tried to claw her way out of the tub.

Both my mom and daughter recovered and healed from their respective hurts, but I was left feeling like a used rag, having soaked up all their tears, pain, fever, chills, and malaise. I was worn and torn.

Parenting a child while becoming a parent to your parent is like being a peanut butter and jelly sandwich. The PB&J (you) oozes out from between two pieces of homemade bread you love (parent and child). It holds the bread together, but it's oh so sticky and messy. The good news is that it is survivable with some kitchen utensils to help you make that sandwich a little less messy:

- Be open and honest about how much you can handle. Know your limitations. Recognizing the early signs of stress and depression can help you navigate this period.

- Ask for help. Enlist family, friends, and local agencies to help. Hire a person to clean house, run errands, or mow the lawn. It is in the best interest of both caregiver and patient to acknowledge when help is needed.

- Take some time for yourself. This is difficult to do when work, carpools, schedules, home care, and children's after-school programs vie for your time. Taking time to do what energizes you and gives you meaning will help you run the marathon that is part of being in the "Sandwich Generation."

- Look for the positive that is in your life, and be thankful for it: a bird singing to proclaim the opening of a new day or your husband bringing takeout home for dinner so you don't have to cook. Look for blessings amid the stressing.

- Pay attention to your own health needs. You don't want to be the person in the TV ad who calls out, "Help! I've fallen and I can't get up!" Instead of the aging parent, you will be the one who has fallen and needs repair. If we do not care for our own bodies and our own lives, we cannot possibly care for our aging parents.

- Don't be embarrassed to admit that you feel stressed or even depressed while being sandwiched. Know the signs of depression: sadness that lasts for weeks at a time, loss of interest or pleasure in activities that once gave you pleasure, a change in weight, difficulty sleeping or sleeping too much, energy loss, feelings of worthlessness, and thoughts of death or suicide.

- If you do feel overwhelmed, stressed, or depressed, talk to a healthcare provider.

- Accept what is, but know it will not always be. This time will pass.

I didn't know all these things twenty-five years ago. I wish I had. Oh, I was an efficient caregiver but one who was a shadow of the warm and caring daughter I wanted to be. I was fried, dried, and empty. I kept my feelings bottled up for fear that if I took off the cap, my insides would pour out in tears, anger, and frustration, and I would never get the cap back on.

My mother's unwillingness to let others help her and my own misdirected sense of guilt and obligation made us miss moments of sharing, with too many words left unsaid. Had I known then what I know now, I would have done things differently.

But I know these things now. And looking back, I could see that God was working for good—not just for me but for the good of others. I believe this was the process or journey that God wanted me to experience so that He could use me for just such a time as this. Twenty-five years later, there I was, walking the dogs and talking to a neighbor who was oozing PB&J while sandwiched between two beautiful pieces of bread.

Surviving and Thriving

While you are the peanut butter and jelly sandwiched between your children and your parents, it's important to remember that you are not the only

Take time to heal and repair yourself

parts that can be used to make a sandwich. Ask for help, and take time to heal and repair yourself. Without you, there is no sandwich.

Prayer

Help me be a good caregiver, Father. Help me use just the right amount of PB&J so that I will not run all out, like a sticky and gooey mess. I know You will help me, guide me, and bring good out of all my circumstances. I rest in Your strength, for You are the ultimate caregiver.

. . .

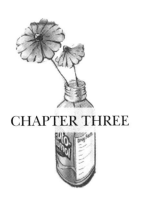

CHAPTER THREE

You Want Me to Do What? Taking Care of Others

3-1. INTRO–IT TAKES A VILLAGE

For I was hungry and you gave me something to eat, I was thirsty and you gave me something to drink, I was a stranger and you invited me in, I needed clothes and you clothed me, I was sick and you looked after me, I was in prison and you came to visit me.

Matthew 25:35–36

As a child, I listened to stories of the lives and deaths of family members. The theme of caregiving was woven through the lives of those before and around me, teaching me that we are all connected and here to care for one another. No wonder I became a caregiver!

In the mid-1940s, my grandfather, a gifted and well-renowned organist, suffered a massive stroke that left him paralyzed on his left side. His sister, upon finding him in such a state, suffered a heart attack and died. It was during World War II, and my father, his only child, was stationed overseas. His daughter-in-law's parents and longtime friends opened up their summer home and brought Pietro and a full-time nurse to live with them until his death. Caregiving crossed family lines.

In 1960, my maternal grandmother was dying of lung cancer. It was a scary time; cancer was considered the "Big C." Being the primary caregiver, my aunt moved my grandmother into her own home. As the lung cancer worsened, my grandmother became bedridden. There was no one to relieve my aunt because no one wanted to come out to the house to provide any respite of care. My grandmother had the Big C, and many people feared catching the Big C. Even nurses were reluctant to come out. My aunt learned how to care for my grandmother, sharpen and sterilize the needles, properly fill the syringe with morphine, and give my grandmother shots to relieve the pain. She had to determine when to call the doctor, what to say, what to ask, when to push, and when not to push. Caregiving was 24/7/365.

In 1980, my mother was diagnosed with breast cancer, and I began my training in caregiving. A year after her mastectomy, she had her gallbladder removed and decided that enough parts had been removed from her body; now it was time to replace some things. The journey to reconstruct her breasts began. It was a long journey of keeping track of her history, how she had to care for herself, and where it would ultimately lead her. She never had any regrets. Throughout that time, I was there to care for her between the surgeries, provide shuttle service, take notes, set up appointments, and help her figure out what was going on with her changing body.

Ten years later, she faced cancer again. This time, the breast cancer had metastasized to her bones. This was a fight she would not win, and as her caregiver, I was there to ensure that she received both physical and emotional care.

More than a decade later, another family member stepped into the caregiving role. My cousin, Nadia, began to care for her mother in 2002. Forty years after her first cancer diagnosis, she developed cancer in her lungs. When my aunt could no longer walk, my cousin would bathe her, dress her, put her in the wheelchair, and take her shopping, one of my aunt's favorite activities. She had a black belt in shopping and a house full of this and that to prove it. She underwent radiation in an attempt to reduce the cancer. However, the treatment's side effect irradiated the side of her brain, which left my aunt unable to do the simplest and wonderfully creative things she had loved to do, such as painting and crafts. During that time, my cousin was my aunt's hands, feet, and brain.

Caregiving was well represented in my husband's family as well. My mother-in-law, Momo, grew up on a farm in rural Indiana. When Momo was only twelve years old, her mother became ill, and Momo had to physically care for her mother as well as cook for the ten to fifteen farmhands on a daily basis. That began a life of caregiving that would span seventy-eight years. She married a man who had polycythemia vera (too many red blood cells) and chronic myelogenous leukemia. She spent twenty years of her life caring for him until his death. She also cared for her parents and in-laws as they entered their twilight years, taking care of each of them as they approached the end of their days on this Earth.

She also cared for her sister, who at an early age suffered from an undiagnosed disease. Her sister suffered from episodes during which Momo would help care for her, run the house, and make dinner. Then she would go home and repeat the same process for her own family. Were that not enough, Momo worked as a nurse and continued her profession until she was seventy-five years of age. She was the consummate caregiver. When Thad and I had our beautiful daughter, Francesca, my mother-in-law came and took care of me during the initial days after I left the hospital. In her elder years, Momo's daughter, Judy, cared for her.

What is the commonality of this long history of people in our family who have cared for others? Is it genetics? A legacy? What is it we all have in common? I will tell you: *love.*

As caregivers, we are the people who write down the instructions given by doctors. We are the ones who file the medical claims, schedule the appoint-

---

We are what I like to call "archive angels"

---

ments, and keep track of what is happening to our loved ones. We are what I like to call "archive angels." We are the ears when our loved ones can't hear. We are the eyes when they can't see. And we are their surrogates when they cannot make decisions. We ask the questions, and we come forth with the energy to find out what is best for those we hold dear. It is a work of love, fraught with fear and frustration, but done as we hope would be done for us.

Surviving and Thriving

We are all connected to one another by birthright, circumstances, and proximity, but mostly by love. We are called to love one another as God loves us.

Prayer

Lord, You placed me among family and loved ones who showed me the way to love and be loved. Thank You for giving me these people in my life and for those I can help and who will help me. May I be an instrument of Your peace and show the love that You have for all your children.

. . .

3-2. CAREGIVER'S TIMEOUT

If anyone destroys God's temple,
God will destroy him. For God's temple is
holy and you are that temple.

1 Corinthians 3:17 (ESV)

Question: Why don't we take care of ourselves?

I am a caregiver. For as long as I can remember, I have been a caregiver. I come from three generations of caregivers. I married into a family of caregivers. I guess you could say my daughter is getting into the caregiving act; she doesn't have a choice. She has the genes.

Being a caregiver can be a good thing. But there's a bad side to caregiving: caring for everybody else but not taking care of yourself. Have you ex-

---

Jesus was an activist, yet He removed Himself from others

---

perienced the total emptiness and exhaustion that occur when you are the sole caregiver for a loved one over a long period of time? If you do nothing to restore your energy, to renew yourself spiritually and physically, you will surely become unable to help those in need. Jesus showed us how to do this. Jesus was an activist, yet He removed Himself from others to rest, nourish, center, and align Himself with His Father. We must follow His example.

Balance is the key to being a caregiver. I have been working on being balanced my whole life. I either work constantly or not at all. I will work on a project till all hours and then put it away for years. I will ride my bike for twelve miles, three days a week, for two years and then suddenly decide it's too hot outside and quit. I will eat healthily for a week or two, feel great, and then pig out till I feel like I am going to burst.

Why is it so hard to achieve balance? Think of a person walking a tightwire, balancing as he moves along the wire. It is challenging. He moves intentionally, slowly, and consistently until he reaches the other side. That is what we need to do.

Balancing all the parts of our lives takes practice, intentional thought, consistent movement, and pacing of our steps. That is what will help us go the distance. That is what will help us be good caregivers.

But first we must be good caregivers to ourselves. Caring for ourselves makes it easier to care for others, but we must schedule a timeout for ourselves.

I remember when my mother used to tell me to go to my room and think about what we had "discussed" and come back when I was capable of discussing the issue in a calm manner. I hated that time. I never knew what to do with myself or exactly what I was supposed to think about. What did she want to hear me say so I could get out of my room—fast? As a parent, I would send my daughter, Francesca, to her room for timeout to change her attitude.

Today I love timeouts. They quiet my soul. Timeouts tune my senses to be in harmony. They calm the chatter in my brain. Whether it's taking a bike ride in the early morning or finding a quiet spot in the house, we are built for timeouts. Whatever you choose as your timeout, ask God to free your mind and body of all thought and deed. Allow only His words to permeate your soul.

Timeouts tune my senses to be in harmony

I often imagine myself sitting on a warm, sandy beach just before sunset, leftover heat from the day's vibrant sun warming my body and soul. I lay my burdens at the water's edge and watch as God's creation of waves takes them out to sea. I offer them up to God because they are no longer mine. Sometimes my timeout lasts half an hour or an hour, and sometimes they last only ten to fifteen minutes. Whatever the amount of time, I am calmer, fresher, and ready to use the gifts God bestowed on me in a positive manner without resentment, fear, and exhaustion.

God has a way of giving us moments to realize that caring for ourselves is no different from learning a new dance or a new language. It seems foreign until you get into it. Then, once you start learning, you realize how beneficial it is, not only for you but for those you care for. Don't pass over what Jesus has shown you to do.

In fact, the best thing you can do right now is to take a timeout and care for yourself so that you can be the best caregiver God created you to be.

See you by the water's edge!

Surviving and Thriving

The caregiver's timeouts are a vital part of caregiving. Schedule them as you would your loved one's doctor's appointments, and don't cancel them! They will save your sanity and that of those around you.

Prayer

Heavenly Father, You have created us in Your image. We are no good to others if we are half spent before we have even begun Your work. With Your help, we will care for ourselves and care for others.

. . .

3-3. THE JOURNEY TOGETHER

Truly I tell you, whatever you bind on earth will be bound in heaven, and whatever you loose on earth will be loosed in heaven. Again, truly I tell you that if two of you on earth agree about anything they ask for, it will be done for them by my Father in heaven.

For where two or three gather in my name, there am I with them.

Matthew 18:18–20

My mother battled cancer for ten years, and I was right beside her during every one of them. In those ten years, I learned a lot about her, myself, and the process of living and dying.

When Mom was first diagnosed with breast cancer, my baby girl was only three months old. Mom came home with a cavern where her breast had been and the fear that her life was over at fifty-six. As her body began to heal, so did her spirit and the desire to be whole. We began to search for a surgeon who would reconstruct her breast. After many doctors' visits, we found a cosmetic surgeon to take on the task. Three operations were scheduled, and a yearlong process began.

Each operation required a one-hour trip for follow-up visits to Miami every other day for the first week, twice a week for the second, weekly for the following month, and monthly until the next operation. It was a long and arduous process for both of us and was made a bit more challenging because my daughter, who was two and a half years old, went along for the ride. I was fortunate that Francesca was an easy and agreeable child. She was a blessing to my mother and me throughout that period in our lives.

What was difficult was when my two worlds seemed to collide. After my mother's second operation, she was in severe pain. I had brought her home to spend the first few days with us, and that's when my daughter began to spike a temperature of 104 degrees. I was running between rooms, administering pain meds and Tylenol, and soaking my daughter in a tepid bath, while trying to determine whether or not to call the doctors.

By Christmas, my mother's body had been made whole. More important, her spirit was whole as well.

She would unload her fears, worries, and sadness on me

Throughout this process, I had become a sounding board for my mom. She would unload her fears, worries, and sadness on me, and I would go home and cry my eyes out from feeling so down. Later, I would find that once she unburdened herself, she was able to go out with her friends and be the life of the party. I had to learn how to be sympathetic without drowning in *her* sadness. The balancing act of being a caregiver became difficult, and I often fought off depression.

Somewhere along the way, I found myself doing more and more of the things my mother was still able to do. When her cancer metastasized to her bones and she was unable to walk, I brought her to live with us. At that time, she truly needed my help, but my years of caregiving without taking a respite had taken their toll; my reservoir of energy was so low that I felt tired, frustrated, resentful, and depleted. I realized I needed help in caring for my mother. We argued about the cost. She wanted to leave us an inheritance, and I wanted it spent on her care. After two months of in-home nursing care, she canceled the help.

So I began the following daily schedule:

- Wake up at 5:00 a.m. and get dressed for work.

- Get Mom up at 6:00 a.m. to bathe her.

- Feed everyone breakfast.

- Determine what we were going to have for dinner.

- Lay out Mom's pills for the day.

- Prepare her lunch and place it in a cooler beside her easy chair, along with her portable commode.

- Make sure the table next to her easy chair was filled with canisters of edible delectables, dog treats (she loved to feed the dogs), her meds, the TV remote, magazines, her glasses, Kleenex, the telephone, and toilet paper.

- Leave for work at 7:30 a.m.

Although this took a lot of thought and planning, the scariest times were when I was not home. Alone, Mom had to navigate between the chair and the commode and back, which is dangerous for someone who is unable to walk. Remarkably, she fell only once, and it was in my presence. I was able to hold her in my arms as we slid to the floor together. She didn't break any bones, but I felt bruised by a feeling of failure. The high dose of morphine made it difficult for her to remember to take her pills, and even though the pill boxes were clearly marked, she often paged me (no cellphones at that time), asking me if she took her pills. I would have to ask her how many boxes were empty and then figure out what she needed to take. I lived in fear that I would make a mistake and she would either under- or overdose.

As the disease progressed, she found it difficult to rest in one spot for any length of time. We began to change her position every fifteen to twenty minutes, twenty-four hours a day. It was grueling, both physically and emotionally.

My husband and I became the only support my mother wanted. My brother and an aunt lived in town, but Mom did not want their help because "they have their own lives." To that, I replied, "What am I? Chopped liver?" Our relationship was deteriorating. I was meeting all my mother's physical needs, but I couldn't meet her emotional ones for fear of lashing out or falling apart. If I let my emotions run loose, I felt I would never be able to put myself back together and care for her.

I was sitting in her room one night, desperately trying to figure out what position to move her into next, when she said, "You changed, Loretta. What happened?"

The tears began to stream down my face. "When you were still able to care for yourself, you depended on me, and now that you need me, I am used up, burned out, and running on empty," I said. "I am so sorry, Mom. You have three children, and you have a sister who wants to help. Yet Thad and I are the only ones you let care for you. When you deny them the chance to help, you deny them the opportunity to be with you, to love you, for whatever time you have left."

A long silence ensued. My mother stared at me with great intensity—as if she were seeing clear into my soul and heart.

Finally she said, "I get it. I understand."

After that conversation, she began to let my brother visit and sit with her on Friday nights—allowing Thad and me a night out. I had harbored resentment toward my brother for not partnering with me in our mother's care. I was so emotionally and physically blocked and exhausted that I found it hard to ask for help. I kept telling him to jump in, which left him clueless. My aunt began to spend part of every Thursday with her. On good days, she would take Mom out for "an airing."

Asking for help provided a great relief for us

Asking for help provided a great relief for us, and my mother enjoyed spending time with her family.

My mother's wish was to die in her own apartment, so we moved her back and began taking shifts. My mother-in-law, who was a nurse, lived with Mom to take care of her nursing needs. I took care of Mom during the day, and my two brothers and husband rotated staying with Mom at night. It was time of sadness, of acceptance but, most important, closeness with my mother and family that I had never experienced before.

Surviving and Thriving

In the end, I learned not to fear death. I have learned to share my feelings with those who are leaving us because those feelings bring us closer together. I have learned to be a sympathetic listener without becoming one with those in pain. I have learned that some people do not know how to help, while others don't know how to ask for it. I have learned that if we keep the lines of communication open, there is nothing we cannot do together. In the end, it is not how we are born or how we die that is important but rather taking the journey together.

Prayer

Father God, even though we often lose sight of You, thank You for never leaving our sides. The events in our lives help prepare us and guide us to You, and for this we are thankful.

. . .

3-4. INSTRUCT OR DESTRUCT

Hear, Israel, the decrees and laws I declare in
your hearing today.
Learn them and be sure to follow them.

Deuteronomy 5:1

I once worked for a tall, athletic gentleman who told me the story of how he tore his knee while playing basketball and subsequently needed surgery. When I first heard his story, I asked him if I could share it. He enthusiastically said, "I would love to share with the world the torture I endured by the loving care of my wonderful wife. The story must be told. I could get sick or injured again. I may need witnesses next time."

At age thirty-eight, Ken tore the ACL in his knee and needed surgery to replace it. The day after surgery, the doctor released him from the hospital and sent him home with two machines: one to ice the knee and another to exercise, flex, and extend the knee because he could not bend it on his own. Ken was feeling loopy from the anesthetic as he sat in the wheelchair while the doctor gave a list of instructions to him and his wife, Lydia. Instead of listening, he was fading in and out, but Lydia seemed to have things well in hand.

Lydia took Ken home and got him settled in bed. She told him he had to be in the flexing machine for two hours, four times a day, and to use the ice machine in between.

"A day's work," he thought.

The first time she strapped him into the flexing machine, it hurt. He couldn't flex his knee on his own, so the machine started cranking and bending it for him. An electronic dial set the amount of flexing and extension his knee was to endure. Lydia stated that the doctor's instructions were to increase the flexing ten degrees every session. Ken didn't think that was quite right. He reminded her that at sixteen he had hurt his knee, and, although they did not have that type of machine then, the physical therapist would manually flex the knee in five-degree increments each visit.

Lydia assured Ken that ten degrees every session was correct. It might as well have been 180 degrees for all the pain he felt. Because he was still pretty loopy, he figured she must know what she was doing.

So she turned the machine on. It hurt, but, okay, it was supposed to hurt, right? Then she went back a couple of hours later, turned it off, and turned on the ice machine, whereby he experienced some blessed relief. About the time he had relaxed and was zoning out with the help of the Percocet, Lydia returned.

"It's time to do the flex machine."

"Wait! Wait just a minute! Every time I am in this machine, we move it up ten degrees?" He was thinking a little more clearly now. He kept asking Lydia if she was sure she understood the directions right.

"Yes. That's what the doctor said," she stated with authority and conviction.

"Do you realize how painful this is?"

She replied, "Doctor's orders."

She cranked that baby up, and Ken was sitting there with tears streaming down his face. By the third time, she had a little mercy on him. "Okay, we will increase it five degrees and then increase it ten halfway through. But it has to be ten degrees by the end of the two-hour session."

By now he was thinking, "Prison break—how does someone get out of this?" He saw the dial on a little remote that would allow him to set it himself, and he decided that at the next session, as soon as she set it and left, he 'would turn it down.

Sure as clockwork, Lydia walked in and set it a third time. "You going to be okay?"

Ken hoped his wife could see the perspiration on his brow and upper lip. She truly looked like she could feel his pain. But he had a plan and a part to play.

"Please, please, don't do this. I can't take it. This is killing me—can I have some more medicine?"

"It's not time for your medicine yet," she replied sweetly.

Despite his pleas, she put his knee in that confounded machine again.

"Please, don't do this to me. I am dying."

Lydia, clearly frustrated, planted her fists on her hips. "Come on, it's not like you're having a baby."

He slammed his mouth shut. He couldn't possibly compete with childbirth.

He couldn't possibly compete with childbirth

But he had a plan. He would moan and groan and make all the noise he could, and when she left, he'd go for the dial!

So he lay there with his knee cranking back and forth, back and forth. As soon as she left the room, he went for the dial. But the dial was just out of his reach! He leaned over and *stretched*! The dial lay about half an inch from the tips of his fingers. He attempted to stretch again. He could barely brush the end of the dial, but he couldn't grab it. His thoughts went into overdrive: "She is evil. She did this to me on purpose. She knew I'd go for the dial." Regardless, all he could do was lie there and endure it.

More icing and then flexing increased by another ten degrees! Ken figured this was his last shot. He thought Lydia had just left the remote out of reach by mistake. She wouldn't do that on purpose. Once again, she reset it for another ten degrees, smiled at him sweetly, and left. Sure enough, the dial was just outside of his reach.

The next few days passed in a blur of pain, sweat, and tears. Every time Lydia walked into the room, she turned the dial up ten degrees. Ken was her prisoner!

Three days later, the doctor called to check up on him and asked him how he was doing. By this time, Ken had made peace with the machine, and his knee didn't hurt as much anymore. His doctor asked Ken how many degrees he was able to flex his knee.

"One hundred ten," Ken said.

"*Wow!* How did you do it?" he asked, clearly incredulous.

"We're doing what you told us to do."

"What exactly is that?" his doctor asked.

"Increase by ten degrees every session."

"Really? That is *not* what we told you!"

"Well, what *did* you tell us?" Ken said.

"My instructions were for ten degrees a session, with a session being one day."

"Oh, my! Doctor, am I going to be okay?" Ken thought he'd never walk again.

"You will be fine. I would not prescribe such a treatment because I didn't think anyone could stand that kind of pain."

Surviving and Thriving

This story is humorous, yet it provides a strong example of the need to interpret instructions properly. Ask for the doctor's instructions in writing. Many times, health-care professionals may not be clear, and in times of stress, we often do not fully retain or comprehend postsurgical instructions. Understanding instructions can alleviate experiencing unnecessary pain.

Prayer

Our loved ones truly love us, but they are just as human as we are and therefore subject to misunderstanding. Let us love them despite what they might put us through.

．．．

3-5. ORANGE BECOMES ME

Do not conform to the pattern of this world,
but be transformed by the renewing of your mind.
Then you will be able to test and
approve what God's will is—his good,
pleasing and perfect will.

Romans 12:2

After all the surgery, pain, and a measure of healing, adhesive tape gone black and sticky should not be what plagued me—but it did. I wanted to eradicate as many reminders of my coronary artery bypass as I could. The adhesive tape was like duct tape that had sat in the hot summer Florida sun for weeks. It wouldn't come off. But if you can get it off, the glue remains on the skin, and then it sticks to everything from nightgowns to bathroom tissue. And even though you wash, the glue turns black, letting all your well-wishing visitors think you don't bathe.

The tape reminders of this procedure were so bad I asked the nurse if the surgeon was trying to cover my incision or mummify me. Once I carefully and painfully removed the tape, glue was stuck to my chest and torso as well as on my hips, thighs, and left leg. Between the cardiac catheter procedure and the multiple incisions on the left leg in search of large enough veins to graft, I had the creeping crud of gooey glue. In short, I was a mess. I tried baby oil, body lotion, paint thinner, olive oil (I'm Italian—we used olive oil for everything), and even Soft Scrub, to no avail. I scrubbed until it hurt, and I certainly didn't need to feel any more pain.

My cousin, Nadia, came by for a visit, bringing with her a wonderful dinner. When I lamented about the creeping crud on my body, she attempted the baby oil and lotion and quickly saw we would need something just short of a blowtorch. She grabbed her purse, said she knew just the thing, and headed out the door.

"Promises, promises," I thought.

True to her word, she returned in about fifteen minutes (there's a Walgreens/CVS on every corner in Florida). Out of the plastic bag came a bottle of Goo Gone. With cotton balls saturated with Goo Gone, she began to rub the multiple areas that were encrusted with the now-black glue. She explained that when she had tile put in her home in the Keys, sticky stuff was on each of her tiles where stickers had been. She got every bit of it off with Goo Gone. She was so proud. But I was no tile floor!

While she scrubbed the tile—I mean, my body—I read the directions: "Pretest on an inconspicuous area." (Okay, I've got a few of those.) "Do not apply to clothing." (That didn't sound good.) "Launder treated items separately." (Do we need a hazmat suit?) "Avoid prolonged contact with skin." (Oh, boy!)

"Ah, is this okay for my skin?"

"Well, I wouldn't tell your surgeon you used Goo Gone on your skin. But I worked all weekend on my tile floor with bare hands and, see, they're okay." She held up her hands.

I wasn't convinced. "But I think I'm turning orange!"

"You can keep the black glue or be orange. What do you want? Look, it's working." She stepped away to appreciate her handiwork.

It was working. Right then and there, I reasoned that since my mother had been a redhead and I have her coloring, an orange body couldn't be any worse than the adhesive tape.

Besides, orange becomes me!

Surviving and Thriving

Sometimes life requires us to think outside the norm, the acceptable. Jesus was never conventional, and He did not always follow man's rules and regulations. We need to be willing to see and try new things. Remember to balance this with wise judgment and thorough research, or you may just turn orange like me!

Prayer

Thank You for guiding us and our friends and family to be there for one another. Let us relish in the abilities and the gifts You gave us to use in helping one another.

. . .

3-6. DOES ANYBODY REALY KNOW WHAT TIME IT IS?

There is a time for everything, and a season for every activity under heaven: a time to be born and a time to die, a time to plant and a time to uproot, a time to kill and a time to heal, a time to tear down and a time to build.

Ecclesiastes 3:1–3

A story was told of a friend who was dying from lymphoma (cancer of the lymph nodes) and was not expected to live more than a couple of days. Family and friends rushed to get to the hospital in time to say goodbye. The doctor told them that once the respirator was removed, their loved one was not expected to live more than ten minutes to an hour.

However, the patient continued to breathe on his own. In fact, he looked better than he had in the previous two weeks. He said he wanted to go home and die in peace. Once settled in his own bed at home, his wife lovingly asked if there was anything he wanted. In a hoarse voice, he said he would love some orange juice.

"You are diabetic; you know you can't drink orange juice," his wife replied.

He responded, "What's it going to do—kill me?"

Surviving and Thriving

It's not over until the good Lord says it's over!

Prayer

Abba, Father, You alone know the time I will spend in this life—just as You know the number of hairs on my head. I dwell in the knowledge that You are the master planner, and I am the apprentice following Your plan.

. . .

3-7. THE GIFT OF A PARACLETE

But the Advocate, the Holy Spirit, whom the Father will send in my name, will teach you all things and will remind you of everything I have said to you.

John 14:26

My husband, Thad, has a gift. It's not your usual, garden-variety gift. His gift is the ability to understand medical jargon and navigate hospital hallways and medical offices that we and our friends and family often find ourselves in. He is able to remain calm through these medical storms without losing his mental faculties–unlike me.

When I received my diagnosis of breast cancer, I was bombarded with such a rush of emotion (shock, self-pity, anger, fear, loss) that I felt like a zombie. Initially, my brain seemed to shut down, and I was simply going through the motions. Thad was patient, kind, and able to think clearly and steer me to an oncologist he believed I would like and was best suited for my diagnosis. He also understood what she was saying, which sounded like a foreign language to me at the time. He listened to my doctors when the numbness of what was going on blocked me from hearing and understanding all the information given to me. With his knowledge and his patience, I was able to talk calmly with him later about my various options and make the decision that was right for me. He was there beside me, every step of the way.

Because of this gift, he has been able to help many people around us. God brings family members, friends, neighbors, and even strangers into Thad's life, and he is able to use his knowledge and experience in the medical field to help them.

The son of a neighbor he watched grow up is now learning to live with the diagnosis of multiple sclerosis. Thad did research on MS and has been there for this young man as he travels this difficult path.

Not too long ago, Thad listened as the new music director at our church asked for prayers for her grown son, who is having sudden-onset epileptic seizures, when he previously was seizure-free. Following the service, Thad felt called to introduce himself to her and listen to her story. You see, he knows a little about epileptic seizures because he sold a drug for this type of disorder. Isn't God amazing? He moves us through our lives and uses all our experiences to help one another. Thad has created what I like to call his "medical support ministry."

In our Christian teaching, we might call this person a paraclete. *Paraclete* is the Greek word signifying "one who consoles or comforts, one who encourages or uplifts, hence refreshes, and/or one who intercedes on our behalf as an advocate." *Paraclete* is used to describe the intercessory role of Jesus Christ, who pleads to the Father on our behalf. In turn, Jesus told His disciples that another paraclete (the Holy Spirit) would come because He was joining His Father in heaven.

We need an advocate in our lives when we find ourselves on the dusty, dirty road of medical issues. I needed Thad to be my ears when I could not hear what I would be going through. I needed him to be my eyes when I could not see what was in a report or on an X-ray. I needed his faith when I was weak.

In turn, when my cousin was faced with recurring breast cancer that metastasized to her lungs, Thad and I became her paracletes. Thad arranged for a consultation with an oncologist he had worked with and whom he highly respected to provide her with an overview of her disease and possible treatments. I went along to take notes and provide emotional support. A few days later, she asked me about something I had written down in the notes, and I confirmed that that is indeed what was said. She stated that she had not remembered it. She had been blinded by her fear and anger, desperately trying to assimilate all the new information being provided to her.

I went with her when she was referred to a clinical trial and even when she had to have a drain surgically placed in her side to drain the fluid that kept building up around her lung. I learned how to drain the fluid and redress the site. I made myself available for anything and everything—on a good day and on a bad day. We shared the highs and the lows. There were days when she took a blow to the chin, and then there were days when she gave a sucker punch right back to the disease that threatened to take her life. In the boxing ring, she was the fighter; I was merely the gloves that made it easier.

We are all called to be comforters, encouragers, and advocates for one another. When you find yourself in the ring or know of someone who is in that same ring, do not hesitate to walk beside them and be their coach, their comforter, and their paraclete. It can make all the difference. Whether you

---

We are all called to be comforters, encouragers, and advocates for one another

---

are the advocate or asking for an advocate, remember you will not be alone, for where two or more are gathered together, God is there with you always.

Surviving and Thriving

In this life, there will be trouble—guaranteed. Why travel it unguided? Enlist a human advocate to be by your side, or be a paraclete to those God brings into your life.

Prayer

How blessed are we to be able to comfort and be comforted by one another! You have taught us through Your words, Jesus Christ, and the Holy Spirit to be there for one another. Let me hear the cries of those around me just as You hear my cries for help.

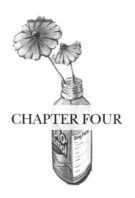

CHAPTER FOUR

What Doesn't Kill You Makes You Stronger: Life Amid Medical Mayhem

4-1. INTRO: DANCING IN THE RAIN

Therefore, my dear brothers and sisters, stand firm. Let nothing move you. Always give yourselves fully to the work of the Lord because you know that your labor in the Lord is not in vain.

1 Corinthians 15:58

During a period of five years, I thought I was in the monsoon season of my life. I tried to dodge the raindrops, but there were so many and they were coming down so hard, I felt I was drowning instead of dodging. I lamented this to a friend, who told me, "God created the shoulders to carry the burden."

"God created the shoulders to carry the burden."

"Well, there are so many of us, God has me confused with someone with broader shoulders," I replied.

We deal with many different and difficult issues–loss of jobs, loss of income, loss of health, and loss of friendships–we feel overworked, underpaid, and overstressed. How do we survive the onslaught? Here are five strategies that can give us strength and comfort.

1. **We must realize that all things work toward good.** Psalm 30:5 states, "The LORD's favor is for a lifetime. Weeping may linger for the night, but joy comes with the morning." God does not promise an easy life,

but He does promise a life with Him in eternity if we trust in Him. That promise has me holding on to the hem of His cloak!

2. **We are not alone.** Cry out to God, our Father! Ask God for the power of the Holy Spirit. As the Holy Spirit anointed Jesus prior to His ministry here on Earth, so will you receive the gift and strength of the Holy Spirit. "You shall receive power when the Holy Spirit has come upon you" (Acts 1:8).

A minister once shared that she envisioned God sitting in a large-enough rocking chair to encompass all of humanity. She could climb up onto His lap, put her arms around Him, and pour out her troubles unto the Lord. What a wonderful vision of comfort! In 1 Corinthians 1:27, Paul wrote, "God chose the foolish things of the world to shame the wise; God chose the weak things of the world to shame the strong." Our faith must remain in God, for as Isaiah wrote, "The Lord gives me power and strength; he is my savior" (12:2 GNB). Armed with God's Word, I am reminded to be strong and courageous, not to become discouraged or terrified amid life's travails. "For the Lord, your God will be with you wherever you go" (Josh. 1:19).

3. **Keep company with others of faith.** We can encourage one another, pray for one another, and help one another as God has called us to do. In 1 Thessalonians 5:11, 14–15, we read, "Encourage one another and build each other up...Warn those who are idle, encourage the timid, help the weak, be patient with everyone...Always try to be kind to each other and to everyone else."

4. **Reach out to those who are less fortunate**. I found myself complaining about the scars I have accumulated over the years due to the many operations and procedures I have had. The ones on my left leg are particularly ugly, and I am sometimes self-conscious of them. But then I thought of my mother-in-law, who in the last ten years of her life no longer had the use of her legs. Then I realized just how blessed I truly am!

5. **Count your blessings.** Even during the worst monsoons of our lives, we can usually find a blessing within them. Maybe it's a friend who lends a hand or a shoulder to cry on or a neighbor who brings din-

---

The thorns may hurt, but the blessings soothe

---

ner when you are just too tired and weak from surgery to cook. The blessings are there for us to concentrate on rather than on the thorns in our lives. The thorns may hurt, but the blessings soothe like a salve from the aloe plant.

Surviving and Thriving

Trouble travels wherever we tread, so don't travel alone. During the rainstorms, remember that you are being refined by God, so reach out to Him. Reach out to community and to those less fortunate. And always remember your blessings amid the storms, for they ease the pain inflicted by the hail.

Prayer

Father, I reach out to You as I travel through this maelstrom. I will keep You close to me, for in You I find my peace. I will remind myself that there are others who are traveling beside me, and together we can forge ahead stronger and more resilient. I will seek out the small blessings that You provide me to encourage me, and I will be a blessing to those less fortunate. I will seek You and find You in all that transpires.

. . .

4-2. CAN NAUSEA BE A GOOD THING?

Not only so, but we also glory in our sufferings, because we know that suffering produces perseverance; perseverance, character; and character, hope.

Romans 5:3–4

When I was pregnant with our daughter, Francesca, I suffered with morning nausea. The moment I would open my eyes, my stomach began to flip-flop. I tried not moving until I ate five saltine crackers.

I tried meditation and deep breathing, but it only sent me to the porcelain goddess sooner. It did not matter what I did or did not do, nausea came promptly upon awakening and left magically at about 11:00 a.m. It lasted for five months, and at times I felt I could not handle it any longer. During a morning porcelain-bowl-hugging event, my husband suggested, "It's all in your head." To that, I replied—well, suffice it to say, I replied, and he never uttered that suggestion again.

A year and a half later, Thad was diagnosed with testicular cancer. He underwent surgery and subsequent radiation from his neck to his thighs. He experienced nausea during those three months. He tried eating smaller meals four to six times a day, but the nausea remained a steadfast companion. One day while he was paying a visit to the porcelain goddess, I remarked, "It's all in your head."

He looked up at me and said, "Touché."

Why one has nausea or how severe it is or how long the nausea lasts does not matter. It only matters that one is suffering. Nausea is real. Whether the nausea is from pregnancy or from radiation or chemotherapy, the feelings are the same. "I cannot continue like this." "Will it ever end?" "I can't stand the smell of garlic sautéing!" "Lord, how am I going to get through work without running into the restroom all day long?"

Regardless of the cause of nausea, one's experience is no worse than another's. At the end of nine months, there is the gift of a child. With radiation, the gift is not as clear or guaranteed. Rather, it is the hope for a long, healthy life. If nausea is the side effect to a new life or a long life, then I, for one, will do what it takes to endure it.

Surviving and Thriving

When is something bad or difficult actually something good? Bad is good when it is a byproduct of creating a life or extending one. Whatever it takes to ensure a long and healthy life is worth a little nausea, don't you think?

Prayer

Abba, Father, there are times when the end results of the difficult moments are good. We thank You for those tough times because they help us see the opportunities and blessings in life.

. . .

4-3. SIMPLY PRAY

Then you will call upon me and come and pray
to me and I will listen to you.
You will seek me and find me when you seek me
with all your heart.

Jeremiah 29:12–13

My friend's husband lay in the hospital's Cardiac Intensive Care Unit with a heart that worked at less than 30 percent. He was possibly brain-dead and on life support, the result of a twenty-six-year battle with chronic kidney failure. My friend didn't know whether to pray for him to live or die.

My friend didn't know whether to pray for him to live or die

Shocking as it might seem, I understood her dilemma well. When my mother had battled cancer for ten years and the doctors no longer knew what to do for her, she knew it was time to relinquish the war. The battles were over. Somewhere during the three weeks it took her to pass on, I stopped praying for her to miraculously live and instead prayed for God to graciously take her home.

As I sat and listened to my friend, I realized that she was expressing those same feelings. She didn't want her husband to suffer. His battle with kidney disease, serious systemic infections, and a weakened heart prevented him from being the athlete he had been in his younger years. My friend stated that her husband had not lived as he wished. If he could, would he admonish her because he hadn't died as he wished? During those ten days that her husband was on life support, my friend prayed that her husband's body would make the decision so she didn't have to. In the end, she had to make the call. When the doctor removed him from life support, he slipped away quickly and quietly.

Living is difficult. Dying isn't any easier.

Living is difficult. Dying isn't any easier. Not wanting our loved ones to leave us, not wanting them in pain, and not wanting to watch their lives be reduced to machines and tubes is like walking a balance beam with no sense of balance. You try to keep your eyes focused ahead of you, but what can you find to hold your gaze?

Gaze on God. The only thing that can hold us centered enough on the balance beam of life is faith. Believing and knowing that God is holding you and keeping you balanced is the key. As long as you keep your eyes on Him, you will walk that balance beam to the very end. Will you put your arms out and walk into the comfort of His embrace—warm, safe, and free of pain? Whether you are the patient or the loved one watching, you can withstand the pain only with the extraordinary presence of God in your life.

Surviving and Thriving

The question isn't whether to pray for life or death. The answer is to simply pray.

Prayer

Lord, I do not have the answers to this life. But You do. Quiet my soul, and let me listen to You, read Your Word, and keep it within my heart. During those times in my life when I don't know what to do, let me remember to lift my eyes to You and pray, knowing You will provide comfort and peace.

. . .

4-4. STOP THE WORLD; I WANT TO GET OFF!

Commit your way to the Lord; trust in him and he will do this: He will make your righteousness shine like the dawn, the justice of your cause like the noonday sun. Be still before the Lord and wait patiently for him... The Lord delights in the man whose steps he has made firm; though he stumble, he will not fall, for the Lord upholds him with his hand.

Psalm 37:5-7, 23-24

When I was young, sometimes my mother would say in frustration and exasperation, "Stop the world. I want to get off!" I think at one time or another, we have all said or thought the same thing. This is true particularly if you find your body doing and going through things that are difficult to endure.

But there you are, enduring barbaric testing and hold-your-breath waiting while still suffering from whatever symptoms or ailments drove you to seek medical attention.

Then you receive the results and think, "Are you sure? Can we do further testing?" Or if you worked in the medical field like my husband and I have, you might say, "Are you sure those are my results and not someone else's?" You experience a measure of disbelief. You seem to be in an alternate universe.

If you were afraid of the testing and the waiting, you find yourself even more fearful about what you possibly could be facing: surgery, chemo, radiation, or death. How do you share this with family when you don't even want to consider it yourself?

Once you begin to talk about it and gather information, you might be like me and tackle it like a work project or home renovation. Are you like a vulture, consuming everything remotely informative about the disease? Or do you just want to protect yourself emotionally and don't want to know? *Just give me the pill, tell me what to do, and I will do it!*

Of course it's not that easy, which is why you want to stop the world and get off. You have to make decisions. People begin to share their experiences. Family members tell you what they want for you. You feel torn between your feelings; your new collection of knowledge; and what you feel you ought to do, want to do, or should do.

I experienced these feelings when I was diagnosed with ductal cell carcinoma of the breast. The oncologist suggested a lumpectomy with radiation. The surgeon advocated a mastectomy with reconstructive surgery. Due to my exhaustive family history of breast cancer, my husband agreed with the surgeon, stating that he cared less about my breasts and more about me living cancer-free for many years to come. It made logical sense, but I wrestled with the decision nonetheless.

It wasn't like I had adenocarcinoma of the breast. My cancer was confined to the ducts. I could always have the mastectomy, but once my breasts were removed, I could never get them back. I remember arguing with my husband: "The surgery, reconstruction, and recovery are major, the result will alter my body, and my clothes will hang differently. You just do not understand!"

"But I do understand. Don't forget that I had not one but two bouts with testicular cancer, losing a testicle each time."

I needed to make this decision with only one advisor: God

Okay, but his pants still hung the same.

In the end, I finally succumbed to the realization that I needed to make this decision with only one advisor: God. I sought quiet time to pray, listen, and rest quietly in the Lord's presence. Ultimately, with God's guidance, I chose the method of treatment I could live with–a lumpectomy. I have not regretted my decision.

Of course, there comes the actual living with the decision(s) one makes. I have experienced an unforeseen consequence to the lumpectomy over mastectomy. Within a year and a half, I began experiencing episodes of what I thought was a rash at first and later learned was cellulitis of the breast (severe infection). I have lived with massive doses of antibiotics, both intravenous and oral, to fight off this infection.

I have learned that such incidences are on the rise due to the increase in lumpectomies. Lumpectomies can cut off the ducts and thereby cause the fluid within them to remain trapped and fallow, thereby causing infection. Once this happens, infection can spread within hours. If left untreated, sepsis can follow. I travel with a bottle of antibiotics. Lymphedema massage and compression garments, along with intermittent antibiotics, have helped suppress the infections. Nonetheless, I do not regret my decision.

I live with the knowledge that cancer could once again invade my body, but we all live with the threat that today could be our last. I work toward living as healthily as I can, each day rejoicing in my life with those who share it with me. I have walked in the shadows of death in the form of braces on my feet as a toddler; removal of cysts, tumors, fibroids ("orchard of fruits," my daughter calls them), and an appendiceal tumor; lumpectomy; radiation therapy; hysterectomy; and a coronary bypass.

I have shouted, "Stop the world, I want to get off!" But precisely because of this walk, I have learned to commit and recommit myself to God, to rest,

---

Every shadow reminds me to turn to, not away from God

---

and to wait for the Lord! Every shadow reminds me to turn *to*, not *away* from God, and it has made all the difference. "Come near to God and He will come near to you" (James 4:8).

I am so incredibly aware that God has been with me throughout my entire journey. I am content in living in the present, knowing that I live with God's arms firmly wrapped around me. The shadows have shown me great beauty, great strength, great love, and great kindness that I would never trade away. The shadows have had their purpose and continue to do so. I look to them as opportunities to search for enlightenment and a continued close walk with Christ.

Surviving and Thriving

So go ahead and shout, "Stop the world, I want to get off!" And then recommit to God, rest in His Word, and wait for the Lord's response.

Prayer

Father God, You have not promised me easy travels while on Earth. I seek your presence more than anyone else. Together with you, I can brave the battles. You go before us, behind us, and beside us. You prepare my way to eternity. Your love will see me through. And that is all I need.

. . .

4-5. MY BODY IS A ROAD MAP TO ETERNITY

Forgetting those things which are behind, and reaching forward to those things which are ahead. I press toward the goal for the prize of the upward call of God in Christ Jesus.

Philippians 3:13–14 (NKJV)

I've done a heap of livin', and I have the scars to prove it. I used to be proud that I had a body without scars. Then at twenty-three, I had two ganglion cysts removed. I put a bangle on my wrist and a bracelet around my ankle and told myself that no one noticed.

Forty years later, I have named my scars after the Florida roadways. The two scars located on my abdomen are I-95 and the Alligator Alley (because they intersect). The lumpectomy scar is a rest stop. The scar from my open-heart surgery is the Florida Turnpike. Three four-inch scars that go from my calf to my upper thigh look like a failed science experiment. In truth, the surgeon had to cut my leg three times before he found a vein large enough to graft to my heart. The first and second veins were too small, but the third was just right! Who knew my body sported *anything* in a size small?

But I have taken a detour from my point. These scars on my leg represent Interstate 4 because everyone knows it's always under construction. I really should lease my body out as a road atlas. Maybe I would spend more time on the highway than in surgery.

Today I am not embarrassed by my scars. They represent battles won. Although by today's standards, my body might look a bit torn up and would not be of interest to any fashion magazine, I look at my body and remember the many things I have learned:

- I can learn about my body and be in partnership with my physician.

- I can persevere with grace and humor.

- I worry less and enjoy more.

- My faith is stronger and my attitude softer.

I place each day in God's hands for direction. Each night, I rest with blessings found in the smallest of visions: the wag of a dog's tail, the breeze on a hot and sultry day. Each day is stitched with the words of God so that this scarred life is less likely to unravel.

My scars are ever-present, a reminder of where I have been. But they do not define me or where I am going. They are a visual list of my medical facts and help me remember that I am God's child, and as such, I can survive anything.

If you need a road map, I am alive and well and living in the Sunshine State!

Surviving and Thriving

Okay, so your body doesn't look like it belongs on the cover of *Cosmopolitan.* Whose does? (They airbrush those photos, you know.) Your body isn't going with you to eternity. So work on what *is* going—your soul!

Prayer

Father God, help me remember that this world may define us by our bodies, but You define us by our hearts and souls. The scars are signs of survival and of continued life through adversities. They remind us where we have been and where we need to be…right in mind, heart, and soul with You—no matter what shape our bodies are in!

. . .

4-6. HIS MIDDLE NAME WAS PERSEVERANCE

Blessed is the one who perseveres under trial because, having stood the test, that person will receive the crown of life that the Lord has promised to those who love him.

James 1:12

Jay was larger than life, with a sense of humor to match. He was a man who did not need much to be happy: a good golf game, a balanced budget sheet (he was an accountant), and spending time with his wife and son. Unfortunately, doctors gave him a poor prognosis to do any of it for very long. Jay suffered from familial polycystic kidney disease—a death sentence he was given at age thirty-two. He began dialysis at forty and underwent a kidney transplant, which failed.

For twenty-five years, he endured four hours of dialysis three times a week. He met, made, and lost some wonderful friendships during those hours, and the dialysis itself was not without its problems. The years of dialysis took a toll on Jay as he became diabetic and underwent a quintuple bypass. What a sad life, right?

What a life indeed! When he was forced to retire because of his health, he served as the treasurer and volunteered to do the accounting for the local Humane Society. Finding homes for "thrown-away" dogs was his passion, and there were always two or more in his home. As he began to slow down, he took up golfing. Even when his blood pressure was so low that he could not bend over to place the golf ball on the tee without fainting, his golfing partner would do the favor, and Jay would swing with supernatural strength. Amazingly, he shot a pretty good game. He just kept living his life to the best of his ability.

He had been told he would never see his son, Greg, graduate from high school. Yet he saw Greg graduate not only from high school but from college as well. He then watched with pride as his son chose a wonderful woman as his wife.

Although Greg readily admits he did not grow up in a normal environment (define "normal," please), through his dad's health issues, he saw first-hand how to turn a negative into a positive. When Jay had his dialysis at home, he involved Greg by giving him the job of rolling the dialysis bags down the stairs to be microwaved. Jay's surgical masks became part of Greg's GI Joe adventures. Even when he was tired from dialysis, Jay would sit on the floor and build Lego cities and organize baseball cards with Greg. Jay and his son created many rituals, such as watching the University of Florida–Florida State games together. When something would happen, Jay would simply say it was "another bump in the road" and keep on going.

Jay used humor as a Band-Aid®.

One Halloween, sixteen-year-old Greg begged his parents to allow him to have a party at their house. They told Greg he could have the party, but only for those he personally knew. That gave Jay the idea to dress up as a cow (udders and all) and crash the party. When Greg opened the door, there stood a silent cow (Jay) waiting to be let in. Greg, not knowing who it was, kept asking the cow questions, but the cow remained silent—at least until Greg's mother could no longer hold back the laughter.

Most people would be depressed if they had to use a motorized scooter because they could no longer walk long distances. But Jay accessorized his scooter with flame decals, handle streamers, and a large horn and would ride through the neighborhood.

As Jay's days became numbered, his cardiologist suggested a combo defibrillator and pacemaker. Jay's response was, "Doc, let's wait till I'm dying because right now I'm still golfing."

Later, Jay's doctor shared with Jay's wife that Jay had taught him how to live and that it was okay to die. He said meeting Jay had been a gift.

Erma Bombeck stated, "When I stand before God at the end of my life, I would hope that I would not have a single bit of talent left and could say, 'I used everything you gave me.'"

Jay lived his life that way. When God called Jay to a "higher service," God met Him with open arms. The Lord said, "See those dogs over there? They are the ones that lived out their lives in love and comfort because of you.

God places people in our lives for a reason

And you have shown your wife and grown son how to live well the life I chose for them. Now go play golf with your friends you met in dialysis. Welcome home, my son!"

Surviving and Thriving

God places people in our lives for a reason. They are angels in our midst. Look, watch, and learn from them.

Prayer

Father, I want to live my life with simple abundance, joy, and humor as I face the pain in my life. May I be a Job or a Jay in the twenty-first century so that I might proclaim, "But he knows the way that I take; when he has tested me, I will come forth as gold" (Job 23:10).

. . .

4-7. NEVERTHELESS

Stay on good terms with each other, held together by love.

Hebrews 13:1 (MSG)

I'm glad my husband didn't marry me based on looks or sex because the only things that look good and feel alive right now are my nails.

I once was a vivacious, voluptuous, attractive woman in a Sophia Loren kind of way. Okay, maybe not quite Sophia Loren, but what I lacked in Italian beauty, I made up for in personality and movement. Ah, but change is inevitable. Gravity has been pulling on this body for almost sixty years. It didn't help that I always felt like I could do anything, including moving wall units, pianos, and curio cabinets. Medical conditions have necessitated numerous surgeries. I've decided I am not having elective surgery until my sagging eye-lids prevent me from reading, writing, and recognizing my grandchild (and need clothespins to hold my eyelids open).

Because my cancer was estrogen- and progesterone-positive, I took Arim-idex for five years to block any remaining cancer cells that my body might use against me. I underwent a hysterectomy to reduce the risk of uterine and ovarian cancer and to remove the "orchard of fruits"—the cysts, fibroids, and tumors growing in my uterus.

After the hysterectomy, I found myself a bit cranky and depressed (that's saying it mildly), so my doctor prescribed Effexor, which I took for six years to lighten my mood. Between the hysterectomy, the Arimidex, the Effexor, and the naturally occurring stress in today's living, my libido moved to Antarctica.

Nevertheless, my wonderful and patient husband still sees the Sophia Lo-ren in me. (I'll admit, his eyesight is somewhat less than 20/20.) And I still see the Thad Schoen I fell in love with. How good is that? Even better is that the love that drew us together wasn't based on animal magnetism. No, our love was and is based on shared morals, goals, and true respect for each oth-er. And so with patience (mostly Thad's, I must admit), we find other ways to demonstrate our love: holding hands, cuddling, sharing mutual inter-

Love can never be surgically removed

ests—cooking, music, movies, reading, biking—and doing projects together (no more moving the piano or the curio cabinet). And if the sparks should ignite—well, it's the Fourth of July!

The bottom line is that breasts and ovaries come and go, but love can never be surgically removed.

Surviving and Thriving

Regardless of what medical issues affect your life, work to keep lines of communication open with your spouse. Find ways to affirm and confirm your love. Let your love shine through!

Prayer

Father God, help us see each other as You see us. Keep us attracted to each other's soul so that regardless of life's travails, the desires of the heart keep us yoked together.

. . .

4-8. THE MEN IN WHITE COATS ARE COMING TO GET ME

The Lord is close to the brokenhearted and saves those who are crushed in spirit.

Psalm 34:18

It had been two months since my mother passed away. When she died, I experienced an array of feelings. I felt relief that her pain was over and that I no longer had to bear witness to it and guilt over feeling relieved. And then there was the overwhelming laundry list of things that had to be done: clearing out her condo, putting it up for sale, executing her will, and keeping my feelings in check so I would not adversely affect my daughter or the other members of my family.

But the biggest feeling was the void in my days where she had been…the

Frightened, Insecure, Neurotic, Exhausted, I was definitely fine!

day-to-day caring for someone I loved more than myself. Oh, I went about my days with all the efficiency of a typical Type A personality, telling myself what I needed to do to get the jobs done. And I thought I was doing well. Mom's condo had a buyer, and I had the entire contents sorted, distributed to family, and sent to auction. I had a three-weekend garage sale and handled all the financial affairs.

I was fine. Really. You know what *fine* means, don't you? Frightened. Insecure. Neurotic. Exhausted. I was definitely fine!

I had some minor health issues during the first six to eight weeks following her passing. Well, actually, it was more like an onslaught! I developed a cold and a yeast infection, and then my face broke out in acne so severe that when I smiled, it hurt. Then came a urinary tract infection, followed by back problems that forced me into an over-the-door traction device that looked like something out of the torture chambers of the Middle Ages. I presented my problems to my internist, whose response was that my body had been in such a state of adrenaline and hyperdrive while my mother was ill that now that the pressure was off, my body was retaliating. I needed to rest and heal. I did rest, and the "disease of the week" syndrome became a thing of the past. I began to heal physically.

Although I thought I was healed from the emotional pain, I found out there was more healing to be done. My epiphany came on that first Mother's Day after Mom's death.

My brother's family and mine were to get together to share a Mother's Day brunch, but at the last minute, they were unable to join us. Following the delivery of that news, the façade of the previous two months cracked and came apart—and me along with it. There is no way to describe what I was feeling except that I was inconsolable, broken, ranting, and raving that I needed family and needed to "feel" my mom's presence somehow. No matter what my poor husband said to try to console me, it just flamed my anger and sent me rushing to the door with car keys in hand. I was driving...but to where?

After some time, I drove to Mom's condo. In searching for some essence that was my mom, I realized that even though this had been her home, little was left to remind me of her. Gone were her furniture, her pictures, and mementos of her life. Even the wallpaper no longer felt like hers—it, too, was fading from life. With the exception of two closets filled with her clothes, the apartment was empty.

I went looking for my mom but couldn't find her. My need to "feel" her was so strong that I stepped into her bedroom walk-in closet and grabbed a group of evening gowns, hugging them as I slipped to the carpeted floor and sobbed. The release of a year's worth of emotion spilled out. All the pain of watching her die, refraining from showing emotion for fear of my

---

With those tears, I was able to face my grief

---

undoing or causing anyone discomfort came tumbling out in what surely must have looked like a crazy person's descent into insanity, had anyone been watching. As I sat hugging the gowns to my body and smelling the perfume my mother used to wear, I remembered thinking, "Gosh, I will never be able to sell these gowns if I don't stop crying on them." And quickly after that, I thought, "If anyone in the building hears me, they are surely going to call the men in white coats to come get me and take me to a padded cell."

I stayed there for about an hour. With those tears, I was able to face my grief and relieve myself of the pain I had prevented myself from feeling. Slowly, thoughts of my mother as she had been throughout my life began to replace the sobs. I began to look at the clothes in her closet and relive happy memories of when she had worn them. I smiled at some of the clothes—her favorite Hawaiian print cotton robe that she would inevitably grab to cover her leopard-print nightgown when someone came unannounced to her front door. Her old white painter's pants and top she used when she refinished furniture. And then there were her eight red wigs!

I began to laugh. My mom would always be with me because I had her in my heart! I had wanted to be with family to be near my mother, but I realized I could "feel" my mother at any time, in any place. My memories and my love would take me to her. In the end, the men in white coats were not called, but my mom's spirit is alive and well in me and in my heart.

Surviving and Thriving

Sometimes we need to visit the "padded cell"—or a closet full of our mother's clothes—to bring healing to our broken spirits.

Prayer

Abba Father, it is just as important to feel our emotions as it is to feel the presence of our loved ones. Releasing our emotions brings relief. Help us remember that time spent with our feelings not only relieves us but draws us closer to You.

· · ·

4-9. A KARATE CHOP SENDS A CLEAR MESSAGE FOR HELP

Ask and it will be given to you, seek and you will find; knock and the door will be opened to you. For everyone who asks receives; the one who seeks finds; and to the one who knocks, the door will open.

Matthew 7:7–8

Buffalo Springfield lyrics are running through my head as I listen to my mother talk with the doctor: "There's something happening here. What it is ain't exactly clear."

My mother lamented to her physician one day, "Doctor, I have been coming to your office every month for four months with the same complaints. Every month, you order blood tests and X-rays and then explain away my complaints and pain with one excuse or another. But I am not getting better. I am getting worse, and you have given me no suitable reason for my symptoms."

"Yours is a difficult case, Mrs. Yon."

"I appreciate that, Dr. H. Nevertheless, I need some answers. Let me show you where I hurt."

With that, my mother steadied herself against the examining table and grabbed hold of the doctor, turned him around so that his back was toward her, and proceeded to point out all the areas on his body in which she was experiencing pain. She looked like she was giving him karate chops to each of his sides, the small of his back, and his legs. I jumped out of the chair because I thought she was beating up the doctor. Exhausted from the energy spent on this demonstration, she leaned back against the examining table.

The doctor turned back around, his face as white as the tissue-paper sheet covering the examining table and said, "Mrs. Yon, your breast cancer may have spread to your bones."

"Well, now at least we have a place to start looking."

Not knowing what was happening had driven my mother crazy. The knowledge of what she might be fighting was preferable to not knowing and imagining what it might be. "Better the devil you know," she'd say.

That visit would result in the diagnosis of metastatic breast cancer to her bones, and she received medicine that helped extend her life for five more years.

Surviving and Thriving

Don't be afraid to speak clearly and ask questions of your doctor. Fear resides in the unknown and enlightenment in the knowing. Doctors are here to help us bridge the language barrier between the medical world and our world. No one knows your body better than you, so if you feel there is cause

---

Fear resides in the unknown

---

for concern, there probably is. With more vigor than you are feeling, pursue answers to what is causing you to feel poorly. If you don't have the energy to do so, enlist a family member or friend to advocate on your behalf. Don't wait, and don't make excuses. Your life may depend on it.

Prayer

Dear Jesus, help those whom You have gifted with healing the ability to listen to their patients, to instruct succinctly, and to use their knowledge effectively without complacency to allay their patients' concerns about insurance compliancy and office schedules. Help us as patients to fully disclose our issues clearly and to question physicians regarding our health issues so that we might be partners together in our care.

CHAPTER FIVE

Living in the State of Joy: A Good Attitude Is a Beatitude

5-1. INTRO: I'M SPORTIN' A 'TUDE!

Therefore, as God's chosen people, holy and dearly loved, clothe yourselves with compassion, kindness, humility, gentleness and patience. Bear with each other and forgive one another if any of you has a grievance against someone. Forgive as the Lord forgave you. And over all these virtues put on love, which binds them all together in perfect unity.

Colossians 3:12-14

The word "joy" can be defined as freedom from want and distress, a source or cause of keen pleasure or delight, inner peace, or a feeling of gladness or the desire to rejoice. Joy comes in many different forms and is as varied as the plethora of people on this planet. It is individual and personal.

Often we think that a new article of clothing, a new car, or a good job will bring us joy. Or sometimes we find ourselves thinking that if our husbands were more romantic or if our children would help around the house more, we would find joy. However, none of those things are lasting; they are fleeting. Author Sarah Ban Breathnach said, "Learning to live in the present moment is part of the path of joy." The only way for joy to be long-lasting is for it to be within us.

STATE OF JOY

By Sally Huss

Some people live in California,
Others in Arizona, New York, or Maine.

Still others live in the State of Joy.
Many wonder how to get there.
It's easy really, requiring no travel.

Simply,
The decision to be there.

. . .

5-2-. GIVE AND TAKE

Although the LORD gives you the bread of adversity and the water of affliction, your teachers will be hidden no more; with your own eyes you will see them.

Isaiah 30:20

My daughter, who was three years old at the time of my mother's breast reconstruction, had only a very basic understanding of what was happening. Although we adults grappled with the loss, the changes, and the public reaction, Francesca took it all in stride. Sometimes when she would have a "slumber party" at Nana's, Mom would get Francesca settled with a project or a TV show and then run a bath for herself. Francesca thought it was time for her to bathe as well and would hop right into the tub with her Nana. My mother, unsure of what to do, decided to act as if nothing was unusual.

On one such visit, Francesca asked, "Nana, why do you only have one breast and my mommy has two?"

"Well, Francesca, my left breast was sick, and the doctor had to remove it. But the surgeon is making me a new one."

This seemed perfectly logical to Francesca, who had often seen children getting new parts for their bodies when she came with me to take her Nana to the doctor.

One particular visit to the surgeon reminded us of the wonderful perspective children have. Francesca was playing on the floor of the waiting room with one of the children. Upon seeing my mother come out of the examining room, Francesca stopped playing and ran up to her with great excitement. "Nana, Nana! Did the doctor give you your booby back?"

The people in the waiting room were speechless—but only for a moment.

Suddenly, laughter came spilling forth from the people in the waiting room and each of the examining rooms. Then everyone in the office suite—patients, nurses, family, friends, and doctors—began laughing as well

My mother's response? "He's working on it, darling!"

Surviving and Thriving

Look with "new eyes" at the issues in your life—through the eyes of Christ.

Prayer

Adversity will plague my life, Father. Open my eyes to the special moment: appreciation of a physician's talent or knowledge, a child's simple approach to life, and shared laughter.

. . .

5-3. GOD'S SECONDHAND STORE

The mind governed by the flesh is death, but the mind governed by the Spirit is life and peace.

Romans 8:6

I have decided that God must have run out of new parts when He was making me. Having lived for more than half a century, I have had ample time to think about this. I am almost certain that parts of me are recycled. I truly think when running out of parts, He thought, "Who could manage with used parts?" And I, obviously, am one of His chosen.

You see, I have problems with the left side of my body. I have decided this is because the parts on this side are retreads. At least that's what I call them. I mean, you can buy retread tires; reconditioned computers; and rebuilt parts for your car, phones, and so on. God, being all-knowing, immediately knew that reconditioning body parts was the way to go. Why has it taken us so many years to learn about reconditioned parts? God must have used them in creation.

Let me explain. I have a bum left knee. I had breast cancer in my left breast. I have bursitis on my left shoulder. I have tingling in my fingers—guess which side? I had to have a ganglion cyst removed from my left foot. When I had my open-heart surgery, they needed to graft veins from my legs. The first and second incisions produced veins too small to use, but the veins taken from the third were just right! (Sounds like the story of "Goldilocks and the Three Bears.") And which leg was that all done on? The left leg, of course. The left hip has been dislocated twice. I am telling you, my left side is made up of reconditioned parts. But it's okay because I can deal with it. I view these issues as challenges to see if I can still function without looking like a Cyclops. Besides, I still have my whole right side.

Surviving and Thriving

It is mind over matter. If you don't mind, it doesn't matter.

Prayer

Thank You for the gift of the Spirit, who aids us by overcoming the flesh and living with You in the Spirit.

.   .   .

5-4. PRACTICE MAKES PERFECT

We have different gifts, according to the grace given to each of us.

Romans 12:6

My husband, Thad, was first diagnosed with testicular cancer in 1981. It manifested with pain and persistent infection of the right testicle. After six weeks of antibiotics and anti-inflammatory medication, the swelling and lump were only slightly reduced, so the doctor scheduled a biopsy, which showed a seminoma tumor. Rather than cut into it, the medical team removed Thad's entire right testicle and put an implant in its place.

Needless to say, we were frightened. Thad was thirty-two, I was twenty-six, and just eleven months prior, we had become parents to our daughter, Francesca. We thought, "People this young don't get cancer, do they?"

Neither of us knew anything about testicular cancer or what the opera-

---

Having an alive and well husband was mandatory

---

tion entailed. I did not care. I was in love with my husband, and we had plans to raise our daughter together, play with our grandchildren, and grow old together. *Nothing* was going to change those plans! I cared for him, not his testicle, and told the doctor as much. Having an alive and well husband was mandatory. Testicles were optional.

When they wheeled Thad into his hospital room after surgery, neither of us wanted to ask exactly what had been removed. The nurse said that as soon as his bodily functions returned to normal, Thad would be discharged. To Thad, that was the sound of the charge, and every couple of minutes, he wanted to stand up and try to relieve himself in the handheld urinal. I did not look, for fear that my face would give away anything that might hurt my husband. During one of those attempts, the doctor walked in.

He helped Thad settle back onto the bed and asked how he was feeling. Thad said he felt pretty good, with just a little pain. Then, in a movement that can be described only as the fast, fluid movement of a bullfighter taunting the bull with the red flag, the doctor pulled back the covers to reveal my husband's resplendent and very naked privates (a complete three-piece set!) basking in the room's daylight.

"Well, what do you think?" Dr. T asked with pride.

Embarrassed and not having any earthly idea of how to respond, I quipped, "What's not to like?"

"I could have given him a small, medium, large, or *wow* testicle. I think I matched his right one with the left one pretty well."

Needless to say, Thad and I were amazed at how noninvasive the surgery was. A small incision that looked like he had just had his appendix out was the only noticeable difference.

Sixteen years later, Dr. T, Thad, and I would meet again so the doctor could remove another seminoma tumor, this time in Thad's left testicle. Dr. T's hair was grayer, and we were fatter, but the operation was the same. However, over time, the incisions looked markedly different. Thad's first incision was wider and still noticeable after sixteen years, while his second incision was barely visible ten years later. When asked why the difference, Dr. T responded, "I got a lot better."

To this day, we laugh when we remember these events. In both incidents, Dr. T had used humor to take away some of the fear that a very frightened couple was feeling. We would continue to use this lesson time and time again as we traversed very difficult medical issues in our lives.

Surviving and Thriving

Make sure your doctor has experience and is well equipped to perform the procedure. Always order experience with a side of humor!

Prayer

Thank You for giving each of us special and unique gifts. And thank You for the doctors who use their gifts to help and heal.

. . .

5-5. SHE'S COME UNDONE!

See, I am doing a new thing! Now it springs up; do you not perceive it? I am making a way in the wilderness and streams in the wasteland.

Isaiah 43:19

My aunt had a strong desire to be the best she could be. She used all sorts of products to help keep her looking as young as she could. The year following her radical mastectomy, circa 1970, wigs, false eyelashes, and acrylic nails were all the rage, and my aunt availed herself of all these products.

One night, as our family gathered around the television to watch the movie of the week, my aunt slowly began to unwind. She removed her breast prosthesis and lay it on the cocktail table. Then she began to work the false eyelashes loose, placing them beside her breast. Then off came the wig and hairpins, along with a few loose acrylic nails.

At the end of the movie, the family began to collect their belongings and say good night to one another when suddenly my aunt burst out in uncontrollable laughter.

She pointed to the table and said, "Be sure to say good night to your mother, children. She's right there on the table!"

Surviving and Thriving

Don't be afraid to try new things. Sometimes they work, and sometimes they just make you laugh. Either way, you win.

Prayer

As we traverse this bumpy gravel road called life, I will remember that I am merely passing through on my way to eternity with You, Lord.

5-6. WE CAN'T—GOD CAN

He said to me, "My grace is sufficient for you, for power is made perfect in weakness."

2 Corinthians 12:9

Have you experienced a time when so much was going on in your life that every event felt like you were being shocked with a stock prod?

There was a time when my husband was working at a job that he absolutely adored. It seemed tailor-made for him. It encompassed all he had learned from his studies and his prior jobs. It was a great culmination to his working career.

But it was getting harder and more challenging to do. The stress level had always been high, but as he began having health issues, his work became more taxing. He was tired. So tired that if he sat in one place (on the couch, at a friend's house, at a restaurant) for only a few minutes, he would fall asleep! His thought processes were skewed, and he was involved in several car accidents.

Then the physical symptoms continued with eczema—just a mild case. But as the work stress increased, so did the eczema. It covered most of his body. He tore his right bicep muscle while trimming some trees in our backyard. He began physical therapy. He also began having sudden-onset diarrhea—cause unknown. Despite seeing a number of different doctors and taking various medications, the diarrhea continued for more than a year. My husband began carrying a change of underwear and a pair of Depends in his briefcase!

One night before giving a dinner lecture, he fell off a steep curb and tore his rotator cuff. At a national sales meeting, he tripped and tore a ligament in his left foot. He had more physical therapy and a stem cell transplant. Both the foot and shoulder showed some improvement but continued to limit his activities. The worst was a rash that began to develop between his "cheeks"—not the public cheeks on your face but those private cheeks. More doctors and more creams and powders, to no avail. I was beginning to think he and Job were related. How he maintained his kind and gentle spirit was beyond me.

I was worried, and I was scared. I would have "prayer meetings" with the Lord, in which I would talk and talk and talk, trying to figure out what was wrong. Because I had a little medical knowledge, I thought the worst, of course: he had cancer, and I was going to lose him. When I wasn't talking to the Lord, I was nagging my husband.

"You need to seek other physicians."

"You need to take some sick days and rest."

"You need to do this, don't do that, yak, yak, yak."

"You cannot keep taking the same medicines and expect a different outcome." Okay, that was good, but it was lost in my drone of negativity.

My approach was bad

My approach was bad. I badgered, nagged, harassed, threatened, and generally made his life miserable. And he was already miserable! He was not at his best, and I certainly was not at mine.

Eventually, Thad realized he needed a lifestyle change. After consulting our financial planner, he learned that he did not need to work up to the age of sixty-seven. So he retired and spent the first four months catching up on his sleep and destressing. The eczema began to recede until it became just an intermittent flare. Thad found a gastroenterologist who properly diagnosed his diarrhea problem being twofold: *H. pylori* bacteria and poor food transportation through the intestines due to radiation treatments he'd had to treat his cancer when he was thirty-two years old.

The proper combination of medicines has resolved that problem completely. The gastroenterologist recommended a proctologist, who properly diagnosed the "cheek" rash. The doctor took him off three creams, prescribed him a cleansing cream, and told him to sit under a heat lamp for ten minutes a day. Voilà! All is clear.

As Thad and I settled into retirement and enjoyed traveling, biking, reading, and spending time together, I realized that all my harassment, fear, and worry had done nothing to help him. I had not acted my best. I asked Thad to forgive me. I went before the Lord to ask for His forgiveness as well. I failed to realize that when I am not at my best, God is at His best. In my need to be strong, I had forgotten that a woman of strength puts her faith in God. God knows what is happening, and He provides for our needs through His Word.

Surviving and Thriving

When we are not at our best, God is.

Prayer

Dear heavenly Physician, with You by my side and in my heart, I am made strong. Help me to not only talk to You but also to listen to You, for You are most powerful when we are weak.

. . .

5-7. WORTH MORE THAN A CART FULL OF COSTCO PRODUCTS

Man does not comprehend its worth; it cannot be found in the land of the living.

Job 28:13

My mother loved going to Costco, but as cancer slowly destroyed her body, she became dependent on a wheelchair for mobility. Regardless, she was determined to stay active for as long as she could. So Mom and I devised a way for her to go to Costco and shop efficiently. I would put her in her wheelchair and find a flatbed cart. Sitting in her wheelchair with me pushing her, she would push the flatbed cart. It took a little practice, but before long, we were like a well-oiled machine. I pushed her, she pushed the cart; I stopped, she stopped. We even got the turns down smoothly.

One day, I parked the van on the side of the Costco building rather than in front, as I usually did. After our shopping was done, we started to leave the building. To return to where the car was parked, we had to make a sharp left turn and avoid the large columns in front of the building. However, the sidewalk in front of the building and around the side was on a slant. (Funny, I had never noticed that before.) As I attempted to turn her wheelchair, Mom tried to turn the flatbed cart.

However, because of the incline and the weight of the cart, she was unable to hold on to the cart, and it began to roll forward into the parking lot. As I saw this happening, I let go of Mom's wheelchair to recover the cart. Mom's wheelchair came precariously close to one of the columns and began veering into the parking lot, too! So I let go of the flatbed cart and grabbed the wheelchair again. Then the cart continued to proceed into the packed parking lot once more. Unfortunately, no one except my mother and I seemed to notice that she and my groceries were about to become chop suey.

Finally, in one last, desperate act of super-heroism, I grabbed my mother's wheelchair with my left hand and the flatbed cart with my right hand. I just hung there, stretched between the two, until a nice man finally noticed our predicament and offered his help. Once she got over the shock of the near accident, my mother started to giggle. She said, "It's good to know how much I am worth—a flatbed cart full of Costco products!"

Surviving and Thriving

Wheelchair: $175
A flatbed cart filled with Costco products: $300
Time with Mom: Priceless!

Prayer

Abba, Father, help me enjoy all parts of my life, even those that seem challenging. Thank You for gifting us with a sense of humor so we can laugh about those times when things don't go quite the way we expect. Help me see the humorous side of life as often as possible. Amen.

. . .

5-8. I'M FINE

The LORD is near to all them that call on him,
to all that call on him in truth.

Psalm 145:18

I have been afraid of needles since I was a little girl with brown Shirley Temple curls and training wheels on my bike. Some things never change. As an adult, I understand the need for shots, immunizations, blood tests, and infusions, but executing any of them makes me break out in a sweat and hold my breath. It brings out the child in me.

Such was the case when I was receiving daily antibiotic infusions for an infection. Although I don't usually have veins that are difficult to tap into, the IV nurse had trouble drawing blood cultures and putting in a new line every three to four days. During the three weeks of infusions, my anxiety level increased, as did my blood pressure. I kept telling myself I was fine–really.

Yup, I was FINE: Freaked out, Insecure, Neurotic, and Emotional.

I was out of control with constant worry. I was so busy flipping out in my own head that I could not think of anything else. "How long will this line last? How long is it safe to keep it in my arm as long as it is working? What if today is the day they can't tap into my veins? Where will they tap into next?" I was on roll into a deep abyss!

Why, after the myriad of medical issues and the plethora of pain, was this fear controlling so much of my heart and soul? Then I remembered that I was trying to handle this all on my own rather than relying on tried and true, practical solutions for my anxiety:

- **P**ray more. Equip myself with the word of the Lord. Habakkuk 3:19 (AMP) became my steadfast verse before and during my antibiotic infusions: "He is my strength, my personal bravery, my invincible army."

- **A**nticipate less. Change what I can, and accept what I cannot. Luke 12:25: "And which of you by being anxious can add a cubit unto the measure of his life?"

- **V**isualize positive outcomes, big or small. I need to visualize the antibiotic decimating the infection. I need to remember that this, too, will pass and that in the grand scheme of things, it is a short time in my life.

- **E**xhale. Instead of holding my breath, I need to concentrate on breathing techniques to help relax my muscles (and my veins). In addition, I use music therapy, reading, and even Facebook as distractions to what's happening.

- **S**urrender. 1 Peter 5:7: "Cast all your anxiety on Him because He cares for you." Have courage and believe that God is able to do what no man can (Eph. 3:20).

Pray, anticipate less, visualize positive outcomes, exhale, and surrender–PAVES. This series of steps *paves* the way to worry-free living.

It was on a Sunday after church that I equipped myself with the above. And you know what happened? Nothing and everything. The infusion went without a hiccup, my blood pressure remained within normal limits, and I was out of there in forty-five minutes flat. As I left the infusion center and waited for the elevator, I realized that God had been with me all along. I burst out in tears of relief and gratitude.

Surviving and Thriving

With God by my side, I am FINE: Faith-filled, involved, knowledgeable, and experienced.

Prayer

When I am lost in the garden of good and evil, I will remember how Jesus prayed in the Garden of Gethsemane. I will reach out to You, my God, my conqueror, and know that all will be well.

. . .

5-9. ROAD WORK

But now, O Lord, You are our Father; we are the
clay, and You our potter;
and we all are the work of Your hand.

Isaiah 64:8

I don't want people to look at me and say, "Boy, she's had a little work done (cosmetic surgery)." You know what I mean. I lived in Boca Raton, Florida, where people get cosmetic surgery as often as they cut their toenails. However, people probably look at me and think, "Boy, she needs to have a little work done!"

I have had work done, just not by choice. I sported braces on my legs from the age of nine months to three years. I have had a lumpectomy to remove breast cancer; a coronary artery bypass to unclog my arteries; left and right hip replacements ; and a hysterectomy to remove bleeding fibroids, cysts, and a benign tumor.

Do you think I would choose this pain and pay to go through it? The thought of having any elective work done is too exhausting for words. So I will live with my sagging breasts that are in a race with my thighs to see which can get to my ankles first. I can live with droopy eyelids–when they are bad enough, I will use clip-on earrings to hold my eyelids up so I can see. Who knows? I might start a trend. I can also live with my basset-hound jowls–they remind me of my favorite uncle and reaffirm that love sees only beauty despite crevices, folds, and wrinkles in the flesh of our bodies.

My scars and wrinkles are great proof of the stories (some great and some gruesome) that shaped me (quite literally!) and made me. I don't want to pay good money to hide behind society's view of perfection when I can embrace my journey and share my story. Who knows, it might just help others overcome their addiction to perfection.

More importantly, the work I have had done is more on the inside of my body than what I wear on the outside. And it's the only work I am interested in. I have had work to help heal some of my hurts, habits, and hang-ups that I used to comfort myself. More work came in learning to love people where they are, not where I want them to be, and to let go of the control I really don't have anyway. I have accepted Christ as my savior and learned that I am a beloved child of God, called and sent to make a difference in the world, not for how I look, but how I live. And by the grace of God, He continues to work not *on* me, but *in* me. I am learning to grow in my faith rather than dwell on the condition of my figure.

Surviving and Thriving

Will Rogers said it well: "Some people try to turn back their odometers. Not me. I want people to know why I look this way. I've traveled a long way, and some of the roads weren't paved."

Prayer

Creator, help me remember that You have made and molded me to make a difference in the world. I will make an impact not by being perfect but by being able to show my wrinkles, sags, bags, and scars as what they are–indicators of where life has taken me and where smiles have been.

CHAPTER SIX

Prescription for Healing: God with Us

6-1. INTRO–GOD WITH US

And teaching them to obey everything I have commanded you. And surely I am with you always, to the very end of the age.

Matthew 28:20

When I was younger, I lived by the phrase "God helps those who help themselves." This created a feeling that I could depend only on myself, and it was all about me and what I could accomplish. I often felt alone.

Life experience has made me realize that even when I thought I was doing it on my own, with my own strength, I was never alone. Looking back, I see God's hand holding me through every trial, each moment of despair. Even as I cried out to God, "I can't do this!" He was showing me that with Him I could endure.

Today I live by several Bible verses that help me remember I am not alone. Even if my family is not around when I need assistance or a friend turns out not to be such a good friend, I am not alone. My family is in Christ, and my friend is in Him. Jesus said, "Surely I am with you always, to the very end of the age" (Matt. 28:20).

When I am faced with an imposing task or a frightening life circumstance, I am reminded of Nehemiah. He was charged with the task of rebuilding the crumbled walls around Jerusalem. How was he to do this without benefit of modern equipment or skilled workers? He had his faith in God, and with God, all things are possible. Nothing is insurmountable. In 2 Samuel 22:30, David sings, "With your help I can advance against a troop; with my God I can scale a wall."

Surviving and Thriving

As we face our walls to scale, we pray that God grants us faith to believe and the strength to hold on to His promise of help.

Prayer

Abba Father, help me remember that while this life wants us to rely only on ourselves, You alone are the only means by which we can surmount the insurmountable and find peace amid the chaos that often rules our lives.

. . .

6-2. ALL I WANT FOR CHRISTMAS ARE MY TWO NEW BREASTS

But those who hope in the Lord will renew their strength. They will soar on wings like eagles; they will run and not grow weary, they will walk and not be faint.

Isaiah 40:31

It had been two years since my mother's radical mastectomy, two years of filling the left side of her bra with an implant that rubbed and chafed. In the summer, she suffered with rashes from the plastic of the prosthesis. They were not made nearly as comfortable as they are today. She was tired of being lopsided and wanted to return to what she called a "state of balance." The surgery had left her feeling lopsided. She was forever readjusting the prosthesis; it never seemed to stay where it should.

When my mother would take my toddler daughter down to the beach, they would build sand castles, walk along the water's edge, and play in the ocean. At the water's edge, my mother would hold my daughter's hands. In doing so, Mom would lean over, and her prosthetic breast would pop out.

I don't know about you, but my real breasts don't pop out of my swimsuit when I lean over…well, maybe they do! But they certainly don't bob on the water by themselves. So my mom and Francesca would play "Bobbing for Breasts." At times like those, my mother realized she wanted to try to make herself whole.

She looked for a surgeon who would reconstruct her breast. This was a lot harder to do than she first imagined. When she had her mastectomy, they removed so much tissue that we could see her heart pounding under the thin sheath of skin that covered the left side of her chest wall. She was repeatedly told that they had not seen this done in about five years, to which she replied that she had just had the surgery two years prior. No one seemed to want to take on the task of restoring my mother's body. We spent many hours and many consultations between New York and Miami to find a doctor who would help my mom feel whole again.

Eventually she found an excellent surgeon in Miami who reconstructed her breast. In agreeing to do the surgery, he gave her an ultimatum: she would have to give up smoking before he would perform the three surgeries needed throughout the coming year. He explained to her that smokers do not heal as well, nor do they wake from surgery as smoothly as nonsmokers do. He told her to call him when she was ready.

My mother spent the hour's drive home in deep thought and prayer. Could she do this? God answered, "You can do all things through Christ" (Phil. 4:13). How would she manage the travel, the healing? God answered, "I will supply all your needs" (v. 19). She was a widow and alone. God rebuked her: "I will never leave you or forsake you" (Heb. 13:5). She was so afraid, and God said, "I have not given you a spirit of fear" (2 Tim. 1:7). She was worried, and God spoke calmly: "Cast all your cares on *me*" (1 Peter 5:7, emphasis added).

By the time my mother got back to her apartment, she had thrown out her cigarettes and informed the doctor she was ready.

The year of reconstruction was long. While my daughter was singing the Christmas song "All I Want for Christmas Is My Two Front Teeth," my mom was singing, "All I Want for Christmas Are My Two New Boobs." That's the honest truth.

Fear was replaced by a sense of supernatural peace.

By Christmas, she was in a state of balance. She was so happy. At the Christmas Eve service, she knelt at the altar and gave thanks for all that God had given her: strength, wisdom, and love. Her faith grew so strong that fear was replaced by a sense of supernatural peace.

Her breasts were merely an added Christmas gift.

Surviving and Thriving

There are times when life is filled with lemons, strong and bitter, and we feel as if we will drown in their sour juice. Given time, patience, and hard work, many a lemon has been turned into refreshing lemonade.

Prayer

Abba, Father, thank You for Your promise to be with us at all times, to show us the way, no matter where we are in life. Help us see You in every circumstance.

. . .

6-3. GOD ANSWERS PRAYERS...BE CAREFUL WHAT YOU ASK FOR

If you believe, you will receive whatever you ask for in Prayer.

Matthew 21:22

God answers prayers, so you had better be careful what you ask of Him!

I spent years asking God to give me strength to lose weight, to help me stop this insatiable need to eat.

I kept saying I could not do it alone. I needed something, anything! Maybe I needed to have my mouth wired shut for a while.

Who knew He'd heard my prayers! Instead of wiring my mouth shut, he opened my heart, healed the hurt, and wired my chest closed (coronary bypass, 2010, for coronary artery disease).

I've lost thirty pounds since then.

Surviving and Thriving

Be careful what you ask for, and be ready for it to be remarkable and unexpected.

Prayer

Father God, You are the ultimate physician and healer. Thank You for listening to our prayers and answering them. Answered prayers are hardly ever in our time or on our terms, but they are always in the most incredible circumstances! We rest assured that You answer prayers in ways that are better than we can ever imagine.

. . .

6-4. THE JETSONS VS. THE FLINTSTONES

Peace I leave with you; my peace I give you. I do not give to you as the world gives. Do not let your hearts be troubled and do not be afraid.

John 14:27

When they found calcifications in my left breast, they told me I also had calcifications in my right. "But they are fine because they've been there for a number of years and have not changed," they said, unlike those worrisome ones that had set up housekeeping in my left breast.

I said, "Now that I knew about them, I want them *all* out, every last little one of them."

So on a warm morning in May, my husband drove me to Martin Memorial Hospital Outpatient Center in Stuart, Florida, where I was to have the procedure. Needless to say, I was nervous. In fact, I was so nervous, we had to stop at a gas station because those nerves went right through my body and out the other end.

Upon arrival, I found myself ushered into a state-of-the-art medical facility. The usual examining table stood in the middle of the exam room. But this one had special attachments and a hole that could be sized. A machine to my left and a computer screen to my right hemmed me in. Once I'd changed into a gown, the surgical nurse explained that I would lie on my stomach and insert my left breast through the hole in the table. My breast would be numbed, which meant the rest of me would not be. The machine would locate the calcifications digitally, and then the computer screen would assist the doctor in putting a guide wire into my breast.

The nurse explained that the surgeon would use the guide wire to encircle the area that would be removed in surgery. Once the wire was placed in the left breast, they would repeat the procedure on the right breast, after which my breasts and I would be taken to the operating room for the lumpectomy.

Technology assisted the doctor in accurately locating and marking the location of the cancer. I was so fascinated by the procedure that I almost forgot it was me and my breasts being infiltrated on the computer screen. But I was jolted back to reality when I was asked to remove my breast from the hole in the table and noticed blood on the shelf below. My blood. I had the sudden urge of fight or flight. For a moment, I planned my escape, but then I found myself praying, "Dear God, I really could use the Holy Spirit right now. I can't do this by myself." Within seconds of my prayer, I felt my whole body relax, and a supernatural feeling of peace came over me. Even the nurse noticed and commented about how calm I was.

The surgical nurse cleaned my breast and then turned around to get some additional equipment for the procedure. She cut several pieces of surgical tape and then reached for two Styrofoam cups. For a split second, I thought, "How nice. She's getting us a cup of coffee," but then I realized that couldn't be possible because they had told me to be NPO (nothing by mouth) after midnight.

"What are those for?" I asked.

"We are going to place a cup over each wire so that they are not jarred out of position while you walk to the operating suite."

Walk? What happened to the state-of-the-art medical center? What happen to the technology? While she was placing the cups over each area, I looked around at all the high-tech equipment that was in the room. I looked like I was in a scene from the future—like the *Jetsons* cartoons I used to watch as a kid. Then I looked down at what the nurse was doing to my body—no, not *The Jetsons*, perhaps *The Flintstones*.

I was sitting on an examining table, naked from the waist up. I had wires sticking out of both breasts. Over these wires, Styrofoam cups were taped to my sides, forcing me to keep my arms raised, kind of like a bird ready to flap its wings for takeoff.

"I am so glad to see you wore a button-down shirt today, Mrs. Schoen," the surgical nurse stated. "It will make it much easier for you to dress."

"You are kidding, right?" I asked.

"Oh, no, this is standard procedure."

"This shirt barely covers my 'girls,' and you want me to add two Dixie cups?"

"Oh, don't worry about that. I have a plan."

Of course she did. She folded a crisp white sheet and draped it around my shoulders like a cape. My look was complete. Ready for my fashion debut, she led me out of the exam room to the waiting room.

"You can have a seat with your husband, dear. I'll see if they are ready for you in the OR."

I was stuck in a weird cartoon dream.

I was not surprised at anything at that point. I was stuck in a weird cartoon dream.

"Is it over?" my husband asked.

"Yes. I am to live the remainder my life with my arms raised at half-mast."

I started to laugh. My husband joined me when he heard my story. I was still facing a daunting surgery. But fear, anxiety, and any thoughts of flight were gone.

Surviving and Thriving

God can provide you with the ability to provide everything you need, whether it is strength, perseverance, humor, humility, or the gift of the Holy Spirit. God gave me all the above when I had my lumpectomy. When life seems to vacillate between *The Jetsons* and *The Flintstones*, choose to find the

---

Choose to find the positive in each event

---

positive, the humor, and the life in each event. Most important, know that the presence of the Holy Spirit can guide you during times of great fear. All you have to do is ask!

Prayer

Thank you, God! You are the great Physician. You tell me in Psalm 55:8 to "hurry to my place of shelter, far from the tempest and the storms." I do so with a whispered prayer, and the Holy Spirit comes upon me to traverse the storm with me. My fear dissolves. You comfort me with Your strength and love whenever I am afraid. Having You in my heart fills me with peace.

. . .

6-5. IN GOD'S HANDS

We went through fire and water, but you brought us to a place of abundance.

Psalm 66:12

Do you need to control everything in your life? Is your need to control so strong that you would die for it? My daughter, Francesca, had this need. The need to control coupled with the need to be perfect eventually threatened to destroy her life. Francesca developed an eating disorder. I did what any respectable, caring mother would do—I yelled, cried, pleaded, reasoned, threatened, negotiated, bribed, and generally created what my daughter affectionately calls "the food wars." Nothing worked, not even eight weeks at a rehabilitation center.

One day, Francesca came into my office, smiling and joyful, full of life. The dichotomy between her spirit and her appearance was apparent. She was so incredibly thin; she looked old and sick. I began crying.

"Francesca," I told her, "you are killing yourself, and I can do nothing to stop it. If you continue this way, you will die."

She replied, "I don't want to die, Mom."

"I believe you, honey, but that is what's going to happen. After five years, I've realized that I can't stop you. No more fighting, and no more nagging. I will just love you and pray for you. I cannot control this. I never could, and I know this now." Quiet tears tracked down my face. "The only one who can make the change is you. And the only One who can help you is God. I pray to God it's His will that you survive this."

Francesca began to cry. As we held each other in love and surrender, we

We both began to relinquish the need to control

both began to relinquish the need to control. We had to accept that sometimes we are not the answer to everything. We cannot do it all ourselves, but God can do what we cannot.

I cannot tell you that Francesca's eating disorder was instantly eliminated in that moment of surrender, but it was a catalyst for change—for both of us. Our relinquishing control and accepting God as the ultimate Healer allowed her to change her behavior and to seek medical attention. It allowed me to have faith in God the Father.

Today Francesca is healthy and has two beautiful sons. In giving control to God, she regained a healthy life and is giving life. She is full of grace and thanksgiving, and she is teaching her sons about God, the great Healer!

Surviving and Thriving

There may be times when you think you need to do something to make it right. However, it is often by ceding control to God that we loosen the chains that bind us and find true freedom.

Prayer

Dear Lord, I know there is nothing You cannot handle. Teach me to relinquish the need to control all aspects of my life, and release the fear and powerlessness that often overcome my soul. I receive relief and renewal through my trust and faith in You, for You are the rudder of the ship that is my life.

. . .

6-6. MIRACLES

Have I not commanded you? Be strong and courageous; do not be afraid. Do not be discouraged. For the LORD, Your God will be with you wherever you go.

Joshua 1:9

I was so tired, yet I did not know why. I made excuses like, "I'm fifty-five years old," "I'm overweight," "I'm going through menopause," and "It's those chronic infections of the breast from my lumpectomy that are making me so tired."

Every day I would begin with, "This is the day the Lord has made. Let us be glad and rejoice in it." But at some point during the day, I would find myself too tired to exercise or to exert any energy, and I would end up lying down and resting. It wasn't long before depression replaced those uplifting Bible verses and darkness crept its way into my soul. I had trouble doing my devotions and found myself unable to count my many blessings. I felt very alone.

Only after I was diagnosed with coronary artery disease and underwent open-heart surgery did I awake with the realization that I was the one walking away from God, but He had always been beside me.

As I spent the first few weeks recuperating, I began to realize and list the many miracles God had sent my way to buffer and protect me. Let me share them with you.

I had been seeing a cardiologist west of town. When I began having the symptoms of malaise, shortness of breath, fatigue, and depression, my husband wanted me to see his cardiologist nearer to us. It meant waiting a month for an appointment, which at the time meant I would have to continue to live with these symptoms.

When I finally did see the doctor, I explained my symptoms and said if it wasn't my heart, then I must be losing my mind. He did a chest X-ray, an EKG, and a stress test, which promptly showed blockages as the culprits. He said, "Walk across to the hospital immediately and be admitted."

"But this is Easter week, and I've waited this long. Another few days won't hurt," I pleaded. "I will go in the Monday after Easter." I gave him a long list of to-dos I had planned for the week.

He studied me for a moment. "You'll need to begin taking aspirin and blood thinners and rearrange your schedule. Report to the hospital admissions by three p.m.—today."

I again persisted in trying to delay the admission, at which point he turned to my husband as if to say, "Is she always this daffy?" He kindly and gently explained the seriousness of the situation: I could possibly have a heart attack, and I would need a cardiac catheter and possibly open-heart surgery. *Whoa!* That got my attention.

Having been admitted to the hospital in my own neighborhood that was both familiar to me and where my family and I had always received good care, I learned that my neighbor, Kim, was the charge nurse for the cardiology floor. It was the first time in years she had been asked to work four days in a row. They happened to be the first four days of my hospitalization. She took me under her wing and not only cared for my body but also my soul. When the cardiac catheterization turned into a coronary bypass, Kim explained exactly why I needed the surgery and what it would entail. She answered all my questions and listened to all my fears.

The morning of my surgery, Kim brought me her iPhone cued to several songs of uplifting Christian music. By the time the orderlies came to take me to surgery, I was "covered by the Lord's feathers, and under His wings I found refuge." Kim uses her work as a ministry for God. And the Lord knew I needed that!

Because I had my surgery on Good Friday, the surgeon who usually performed this operation was on vacation. The surgeon on call, who operated on me, routinely performed coronary artery bypass surgery without using the heart and lung machine. That reduced my recovery time and allowed me to go home sooner.

Surviving and Thriving

I realize that God was with me throughout this whole process. He protected me from a heart attack for all those months. He used doctors, nurses, and even my husband to place me where I needed to be, to hear what I needed to hear, and to heal not just my blocked heart but my darkened soul. Those are miracles!

Prayer

Abba, Father, You pave our lives with miracles and lessen our fears with blessings in our circumstances. Thank You, Father, for allowing us to be witnesses of Your love.

. . .

6-7. TALENT BORN FROM TRIBULATIONS

You will again obey the Lord and follow all his commands I am giving you today.

Deuteronomy 30:8

My Aunt Dot was diagnosed with breast cancer at the age of thirty-eight. She was given six weeks to six months to live. But my aunt didn't agree with the professionals. She told them that she had two teenage daughters, and one was driving her crazy. Her daughters needed their mother, and she needed to raise them. She didn't have time to die.

She was sent home with a Kotex pad stuffed in her bra and told to get her affairs in order. She did just that. She researched (this was the 1960s, no computers—just the library) all she could on the advances in breast cancer. She made appointments with all types of physicians, including ones who saw patients only in the middle of the night. Okay, that was weird. But she was relentless in her pursuit of healing. In 1968, she became an expert at breast cancer recovery.

One thing they told her was to exercise her arm to reduce atrophy. So my aunt began to paint. She thought the up-and-down, back-and-forth motions of the brushstrokes would help. Indeed, the painting helped provide mobility.

What she didn't count on was how God would bring out the artistic talent He had given her. She began to flourish. Without the benefit of classes, she used her gift to heal herself and to bring beauty to those who viewed her paintings. Her use of colors and settings would soon be seen throughout the Long Island–New York area. On a trip to Florida, an art gallery in Boca Raton, Florida, expressed interest in featuring her as an artist. She donated many of her paintings to raise funds for cancer research and other worthwhile causes.

Little did she know when she was diagnosed with breast cancer and told she was dying that a new life and adventure would be created. My aunt lived

---

Through adversity, God provides us with new avenues of living.

---

to seventy-three years of age, and she continued to paint until the last three months of her life. Her paintings are a reminder to me that through adversity, God provides us with strength and new avenues of living.

Surviving and Thriving

In pain, suffering, and healing, new life forms are created within us. The journey, although difficult, strengthens us and shows us that throughout all our tribulations, God works to create good in them.

Prayer

Lord, help us have faith that no matter what happens to us in this life, You will be there. You will lead us to quiet, still waters where we can see the good and the new that spill forth from the adversity in our lives.

. . .

6-8. KNOW WHEN TO HOLD 'EM AND WHEN TO FOLD 'EM

Cast your cares on the Lord and He will sustain you. He will never let the righteous be shaken.

Psalm 55:22

"Doctor, is there anything else we can try?" my mother asked during a doctor's visit.

The doctor shook his head. "I'm afraid we have run out of options, Mrs. Yon."

After a ten-year battle with cancer, there were no more protocols, trials, or medicines to combat the disease that was destroying my mother's body.

As I settled her in the car, she said, "Take me home."

"That's where I am going, Mom."

"No, I want to go to my apartment."

"Mom, you can't walk. You cannot stay alone in your apartment. You need to stay with us."

"I want to go to my home—"

"Mom," I interrupted. "You can't."

"Look, I'm tired of fighting, but I'm not afraid of dying. I will not die in your house. I will not die in front of my granddaughter! I am going home, even if I have to crawl over Fortieth Street Bridge to do so!" Her voice was developing a crescendo with each statement.

With that we fell silent, but we were both thinking about how we could make this last chapter of her life go as calmly and smoothly as she would like. Slowly we developed a plan.

We called the medical supply company and ordered a hospital bed, a portable commode, and other equipment to be moved to her apartment. The chemo nurse who had befriended my mom helped us do hospice at home. She visited us in the morning before her shift and in the evening at the end of her shift. She taught us how to adjust the dosage of morphine, change the morphine bags, hang the "Do Not Resuscitate" sign on the kitchen fridge, and change the catheter bag. My husband called his mom, who was a retired nurse. She came to live with my mom for what was to be the last three weeks of her life. I called my brothers, and they and my husband took turns sitting with my mom at night. My aunt came over daily to sit with Mom between 8:00 and 10:00 a.m. I covered the days with my mother-in-law.

After we'd made the arrangements and settled Mom in her apartment, she gathered my brothers and me in her room.

"I want you to know that I appreciate all you are doing for me," she said. "I know you want me to continue to try. But after ten years, I know when my body has said 'enough.' It is now. I have won a lot of battles, but I cannot win this war. Your lives are still ahead of you, and you have some battles of your own to win. I suggest you unload this apartment as fast as you can. The buildings in this complex are old, and being on the ocean, they are in constant need of repair. I have barely been able to keep up with all the assessments. So take your best offer and dump it. Decide what stuff you want, and sell off the rest. I sure don't need it."

She released a sigh before she continued. "My affairs are in order, and Loretta knows exactly what to do. Now you do what you want, but these are my thoughts about it all. I am ready. I've had a full and interesting life. I have no regrets. I do not ask for more." She rested her head on the pillow and quickly dozed off.

As we tiptoed out of her room, none of us said a thing. We never discussed the conversation, but three weeks later, Mom passed away slowly, quietly, and just as she wanted. We followed her advice then, and now we follow her example of a life lived with God and the lessons she learned and shared with us.

Surviving and Thriving

Know when to fight and when not to. Know when to hold 'em, and know when to fold 'em. Sometimes we need to change our thinking, pace, or routine to remain on course with God. Be mindful of *His* voice speaking to you, even when faced with something new and unknown. It takes courage, but "The one who calls you is faithful and will give you the grace that is needed" (1 Thess. 5:24).

Prayer

Thank You, Lord, for giving us the ability to sense when You are calling us home to You. We will prepare ourselves and our loved ones for this time; remember the sweet times shared and the courage, lessons, and faith amassed during our journey together; and rejoice in the knowledge that a new eternal life with You is just around the corner.

. . .

6-9. THE HEALER'S GIFTS OF GRACEFUL HEALING

The righteous may have many troubles, but the
LORD delivers him from them all.

Psalm 34:19

As I get older, so much is going on inside me that I find myself weary before I have even started the day. First, just getting out of bed can bring on the reminder that I can no longer do what I used to do when I was in my twenties, thirties, or even forties. I should have thought of that before I rearranged furniture in the living room (including the piano). But I digress.

Then as I wash my face and brush my teeth, my brain begins to focus on the needs of the day. That can be a challenge in itself—just trying to re-member not to forget what I need to do. I haven't even made it out of the bedroom, and I know I cannot continue without aid to face the day. So the prayers begin. I really want to jump right to the supplications (requests), but I remember all the good that God has done in my life; thus, my gratitude and adoration begin. Realizing the majesty, enormity, and graciousness of God, I begin to recognize my weaknesses, and I confess my failings to Him

However, somewhere during my laundry list of sins, I begin to see the many blessings that were intertwined with my dirty laundry. I realize that with every pain, with every "no," there has been a gain, a joy, a "yes"! Then I petition God to help the others on my prayer list as He has helped me. I will repeat this journey as I begin each day, for this process helps me heal physically and emotionally.

When we think of healing, we think of two types: physical and emotional. Although these are certainly central to our living, they are only two of the five types of healing available to us.

Divine healing is immediate, lasting, and verifiable, and all the glory goes to God. This healing occurs during times when diseases are incurable. The New Testament is filled with stories in which Christ healed the sick, the lame, and the demon-possessed. Divine healing is what most people pray for when their loved ones are suffering from an incurable disease or near-fatal accident. When divine healing has taken place, people often don't believe it or search for a plausible explanation.

God created the world, and *natural healing* is found in all plant, animal, and human life. Yet most of us take for granted a skin abrasion that goes away on its own or a cold fought off by the body's natural defenses and immune

---

What amazing bodies we have!

---

system. What amazing bodies we have! So many germs and so many diseases lurking, yet God has given us the immune system that counterattacks more often than we know. Natural healing may be slow, and may or may not last, and the immune system can be so compromised that without outside help (medicines,) it cannot efficiently heal itself. Today we are so conditioned to give credit or seek out medicines to resolve a medical dilemma that we seldom give God the glory for creating our bodies and the world around us to assist in the repair. God works through natural healing as well as through man's ability to use natural and man-made resources.

Medical healing is obtained by the use of plants, herbs, and other substances God created for our use. God has given humans intelligence, ability, and wisdom to apply learned healing that is constantly passed down and enhanced to help humankind. God often uses medical healing to heal people, particularly in answer to prayer for wisdom for medical practitioners to know how to treat the problem.

Psychological healing is the healing of attitude. The Bible gives many examples of this type of healing. We read in 2 Corinthians 12:8–10, "Three times I pleaded with the Lord to take it away from me. But he said to me, 'My grace is sufficient for you, for my power is made perfect in weakness.' Therefore I will boast all the more gladly about my weaknesses, so that Christ's power may rest on me. That is why, for Christ's sake, I delight in weaknesses, in insults, in hardships, in persecutions, in difficulties. For when I am weak, then I am strong."

Author Sarah Ban Breathnach began her journey to find a balance in her life among her wants, work life, needs, and desires. What she found were six spiritual principles that became catalysts for a happy life: gratitude, simplicity, order, harmony, beauty, and joy. Notice that they are built on attitude. A positive attitude toward your life, your body, and your loved ones is necessary for psychological healing.

The final type of healing is *death*. Death is the ultimate healer. We become healed body, mind, and soul when we join our Creator: Father, Son, and Holy Spirit. Romans 8:17–19 reminds us, "Now if we are children, then we are heirs of God and co-heirs with Christ, if indeed we share in his sufferings in order that we may also share in His glory. I consider that our present sufferings are not worth comparing with the glory that will be revealed in us."

We often don't think of death as a process in healing; however, in death we are truly and eternally healed from all our afflictions. This thought provides me with much comfort as I traverse my days on this Earth. How wonderful is God to give us all we need through plant, animal, and human life, and then when this chapter on Earth is over, another life of infinite, indescribable, magnificent grandeur begins! While I do all I can to allow my body to use its natural healing abilities, use the gifts God has given me to promote medicinal healing, and live psychologically soundly, I know that in the end, death will be the ultimate healer, and I will rest safely in the ultimate Healer's embrace.

Surviving and Thriving

Life encompasses *all* five types of healing, and we must work to investigate, learn, practice, and pray for the wisdom to use each of them.

Prayer

Father of all life, I thank You for providing us the tools necessary for our journey to eternity. I will embrace each event in my life, whether a joy or a sadness, so I might give thanks and praise.

. . .

6-10. DEATH...WHAT A WONDERFUL WAY TO EXPLAIN IT

A sick man turned to his doctor as he was preparing to leave the examination room and said, "Doctor, I am afraid to die. Tell me what lies on the other side."

Very quietly, the doctor said, "I don't know..."

"You don't know? You're a Christian man and don't know what's on the other side?"

The doctor was holding the handle of the door; On The Other Side came a sound of scratching and whining, and as he opened the door, a dog sprang into the room and leaped on him with an eager show of gladness.

Turning to the patient, the doctor said, "Did you notice my dog? He's never been in this room before. He didn't know what was inside. He knew nothing except that his master was here, And when the door opened, he sprang in without fear. I know little of what is on the other side of death, But I do know one thing... I know my Master is there, and that is enough."

Author Unknown

. . .

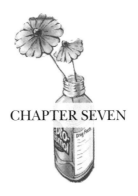

CHAPTER SEVEN

Just the Facts, Ma'am: Keeping Current

7-1. INTRO–WHO IS AT THE HELM OF THIS SHIP?

Your attitude should be the same as
that of Christ Jesus.

Philippians 2:5

I had been receiving antibiotic infusions for ten days and had not seen a doctor since that first late afternoon, when I presented to his office with cellulitis of the breast. I was feeling like a cow that was brought in to be milked daily. The IV nurses were wonderful; they know what they are doing. I had met some nice people who were, like me, receiving treatment for one type of infection or another. Dutifully, we came in at our appointed times and got "hooked up and juiced." We'd chat, commiserate, wish each other good health, and share our hopes of getting and feeling better.

But I wondered: when was I going to see a doctor, get the results of my blood cultures, and find out how long was I going to need treatment.

I was initially told that the doctors see infusion patients once a week, and I would see the doctor on the following Monday. Monday came, but there were no doctors in sight, and the front-desk staff said everyone was going to be seen on Tuesday. Tuesday turned out to be my sprint from one doctor to another and then turned into an afternoon marathon at one doctor's office, which made it impossible to get my infusion before 4:00 p.m., let alone see the infusion doctor. Then I was told I would see the doctor on Wednesday.

On Wednesday, after inquiring about seeing the physician for my weekly update, the front-desk receptionist stated that doctors are not in on Wednesday, but I would see a doctor on Thursday. Thursday, there was a doctor in the office, but he did not see infusion patients! At that point, I offered to go over to their other office if it meant being able to see a doctor. The receptionist informed me that although I could go to the other office, there was no guarantee that I would be seen. It was Friday before I saw a new emergency physician covering for the six-member practice.

Really?!?

As a patient, I work hard at getting well. That means following the advice of my health-care providers, be it the nurses, the doctors, or the front-desk staff. Louisa May Alcott said, "I am not afraid of the storms, for I am learning how to sail my ship." So I am listening and learning.

As a retired medical secretary and a lifelong member of the unofficial college of health-care learning, I could see how this office failed to provide quality of care. The front desk either did not have the doctors' schedules,

---

An informed patient is a compliant patient

---

or they were failing to accurately inform patients of the schedule or changes in it. This was unfortunate because an informed patient is a compliant patient. And a compliant patient produces a calmer office. An uneducated, uninformed patient is like a bomb without a timer that could blow up at any time. Aw, heck, I could have blown at any time!

While each day's antibiotic infusion made the infection look less inflamed, fired up, and painful, my not being informed had increased my blood pressure to an alarming rate. I had the feeling that I was on a ship in a storm with no one at the helm.

So who was at the helm of this ship?

Ultimately, I was.

I thought about it and realized that I needed to do the following:

- Continue an open and respectful dialogue with the front desk, probing, asking questions, and making my requests known. Be specific and clear about what I need.

- Consider that the front-desk receptionists may not be informed and may feel overwhelmed and caught between the doctors and the patients.

- The front-desk staff take a lot of abuse from patients who are not feeling well and doctors who are overwhelmed with work. They may be burnt out and may have disengaged. Yet as a patient, I am a consumer and have a right to know and understand what therapies are being done.

- Speak to the practice manager, who runs the day-to-day operations of the practice. He or she may be unaware of the problem, and my input may provide an opportunity to resolve a matter that is systemic and not just happening to me. In this situation, the practice manager was mainly in the other office, which may have been part of the problem.

- Request to see the doctor, and ask him or her to spend a little time explaining the course of treatment or lack of treatment and what I need to feel confident in my care. Make my requests respectful, specific, and clear.

- Finally, if after I take the above measures, there remains a lack of confidence in the physician and the practice, it is time to request a copy of my chart and seek health care elsewhere.

Surviving and Thriving

It's important to realize that while we, as patients, are learning to sail our ships through the storms of illness, we can be teachers to our health-care providers by expecting the same respect we give to them. We must be the captains of our own ships and steer ourselves through the often choppy seas of health care.

Prayer

In this world of ever-changing health care, I must be willing to man my ship with all I can to honor You, Lord. I ask for guidance, wisdom, and patience to weather the stormy seas. I turn to You for constant direction, for You are truly at the helm of this ship. Amen.

. . .

7-2. DOCTOR SHOPPING

I've heard about you, that a spirit of the gods is in you and that you have insight, discernment, and extraordinary wisdom.

Daniel 5:14

Although I enjoy shopping when I need to, it's not something I want to do every day. I don't have the bank account for it, nor do I need much to make me happy these days. So imagine my surprise when I realized I was going to need a black belt in shopping to find an orthopedic surgeon to replace my hip.

I began by writing down what I was looking for in a surgeon: someone with the moral strength and character of Moses, the patience of Job, the wisdom of King Solomon, and the kindness of Jesus. I was looking for someone who would use his or her education and God-given gifts with precision and skill to do a simple routine hip replacement. Is that so much to ask for?

I began the usual way: asking friends, family, colleagues, and medical professionals about possible candidates. I checked out the doctors' training, inquired about hospital affiliations, asked about insurance coverage, and checked credentials.

One surgeon came highly recommended from several friends. But when I called to make an appointment, it turned out that he only did knees. And although my knees can't get me back up from a squatted position, they still work, and I am not ready to trade them in yet.

A friend of mine who has worked in many areas of the hospital told me emphatically that Dr. So-and-So is the best with hips, but he has been known to have alcohol on his breath. "No worries," she said. "He can do the procedure with his eyes closed, and the nurse practitioner follows you after surgery anyway." Really!?!

Another surgeon operates on hips and does other procedures but not as often as the surgeon with alcohol on his mind–I mean breath. Sorry, Doc, I'm a little too old for a test drive.

Then there was one who was good but treated only what concerned his area of expertise, not the whole person. During one such case, the surgeon wanted the patient discharged despite the concerns from the nurse that the patient was in distress. The doctor was adamant that the patient was fit for discharge–until the patient had a heart attack. Next doctor candidate, please!

I got two names from my physical therapist and checked out their credentials and websites. Both appeared equally impressive. One works with many athletes and 95 percent of the time uses a newer method called "anterior hip replacement." He touts its ease of healing, the fact that it is less invasive, and a shorter hospital stay. That sounded great!

The other no longer uses the anterior method and made a strong case against its use (limited types of prosthetic devices, can leave residual numbness, etc.). The posterior hip replacement is tried and true and has evolved to a point of optimum success.

Can I see the surgeon behind door number 3, please?

After months of networking all avenues of discovery, a name kept coming up in conversations. A consultation with him and his office staff confirmed that I had chosen the best doctor for my hip replacement. My new hip and I are getting along famously, thanks to Dr. L. This is very good indeed because my right hip is going to need replacing soon as well!

Surviving and Thriving

Take time to shop for the doctor who has the most experience, a good "bedside manner," and patience for whatever your needs are. Remember the old adage, "Act in haste, repent at leisure."

Prayer

Father, guide me to be open to all methods of research so that I may be equipped to choose physicians who will treat me as You would want us to treat one another–with love and kindness. Provide me with discernment and patience for this journey as I find the physicians who practice their gifts with You in their hearts.

. . .

7-3. ARE WE CARING FOR THE PATIENT OR

THE HEALTH-CARE SYSTEM?

Do you not know that you are a temple of God and that the Spirit of God dwells in you?

1 Corinthians 3:16

An old nemesis visited me—one I knew well but had not battled for five years. Cellulitis of the breast due to a lumpectomy in 2003 came roaring into my body, and within a matter of two hours had created a 102-degree fever; chills that left me shaking uncontrollably; muscles painfully contracting; and the left side of my torso hot, heavy, and hard. I was in trouble with a familiar foe that left me stunned at the sudden and quick attack.

If you are not familiar with cellulitis, it is a bacterial infection that, left untreated, can quickly escalate to sepsis (a potentially life-threatening, whole-body response to infection). As instructed, I keep a stock bottle of antibiotic in the house or with me during my travels and immediately started a dose. But the night was long, and I knew I had to get in touch with my infectious-disease (ID) physician to get on an IV infusion of antibiotics as soon as possible.

That's when the trouble started.

At 9:00 a.m. the following morning, I called the office and explained my plight. I was told that because I had not been to the office in almost five years, I would need to see my general practitioner (GP) first. Thinking the receptionist was speaking about health insurance coverage and needing a referral, I told her my insurance did not require a referral. Nevertheless, the doctor would not see me until I was referred. Folks, for future reference, this means that they have put your medical record in storage (*Am I dead yet?*), and someone needs to go get it.

156

Being too weak to argue, I phoned my GP and was given a 2:00 p.m. appointment. When I showed up at the GP's office, they took one look at my hot, heavy, and painful breast and told me, "You need to be admitted to the hospital and begin antibiotics!"

Haven't I been saying that?

I explained that this had happened before (the GP had never seen me for this) and that what I needed was an IV antibiotic, which could be administered as an outpatient. Would she call my ID physician? A deal was worked out that if the ID physician could see me and administer the IV, I would be spared a hospital admission, but if not…

At 4:00 p.m., the ID physician did indeed see me and ordered the IV antibiotic to be administered immediately.

But not before I shared my opinion.

Our system is no longer practicing medicine but is managing patients like cattle through a system we call health care. It's more about the care of the health-care system with its standards of practice, procedures, and protocols than it is about patient care. We have given up caring for the patient in lieu of caring for a system.

I explained to the ID physician that I could have been there a whole lot sooner but had been put off by the office staff. Now, at almost 5:00 p.m., after being charged for two office visits, I was finally receiving the care I needed. In addition, I told him that the cost of treatment was now increased because of paying overtime to an IV nurse who didn't need to take more time away from her family–all because the receptionist didn't ask the physician for guidance but empirically decided that I was to be treated as a new patient. One size does not fit all, folks!

The ID physician's response was that they would speak with the front-desk staff but that I could have gone to the emergency room for treatment. If I had not known what was happening or what needed to be done, had not had the oral antibiotics, or did not know how to do it without costing me or the insurance company thousands of dollars, I would have. But let's assume that we all just went to the emergency room for whatever our needs were because we no longer have access to our physicians. We would no longer need the private practice physicians, would we? It seems as though health care is leading in that direction.

In defense of physicians, practicing in today's health-care system is like walking a tightrope without being able to use your arms for balance. Difficult at best. The health-care protocols and practices in our medical system were created without much physician input, and the system is not oriented to good patient care. It has been transformed from doing what is best for the patient to a focus on dollars and cents and cost-effectiveness. Physicians are caught in a system in which they don't have the freedom to practice medicine or to adhere to their Hippocratic Oath.

Surviving and Thriving

We must remind all health-care providers of a phrase that appears in the Hippocratic Oath, which many medical schools still use today: that there is "an art to medicine as well as science, and that warmth, sympathy, and understanding may outweigh the surgeon's knife or the chemist's drug."[3] We must view ourselves as consumers shopping for the best quality care possible because our lives may depend on it.

Prayer

Lord, we desperately need to pray for our health-care providers–doctors, nurses, and emergency medical staff–as well as for change in our health-care system. We also pray for ourselves as people and patients. Provide us with the wisdom to empower and educate ourselves with the knowledge of health-care practices today and to be in partnership with our health-care providers.

. . .

7-4. YOUR MEDICAL TREE

You will be protected from the lash of the tongue,
and need not fear when destruction comes.

Job 5:21

My husband, Thad, and I met in 1973 and quickly discovered we had a lot in common. We were the babies in our respective families, with two older siblings. Each family had two boys and a girl. Both of us had lost our fathers at a very young age (me at age fourteen and Thad, eight), which culminated in our mothers moving to Florida. Our fathers died at the same age and in the same month.

What we did not have in common was that although I knew quite a bit about my father's medical history, Thad did not. So once Thad and I became serious, it wasn't long before I found myself asking necessary questions.

I come from a highly spirited Italian family in which anything and everything is discussed freely at the dinner table, to the point of either hilarity or humility. On the other hand, my husband comes from a quiet German family where the dinner hour was spent quietly eating. Imagine! No discussion, no prodding, no provoking, no questioning—just pleasantly eating the evening's repast. Out of respect for their mother, no one in Thad's family had discussed his father's medical history. They did not want to upset her. That is, until I came and broke the silence.

Picture this: It's 1974, and I am visiting my future mother-in-law. I awaken to the wonderful aroma and sounds of breakfast preparation. I pad out and offer to set the table for her, and I begin to do what comes inherent to me–I ask her about her husband, their life, and his illness and eventual death. Unknown to me, Thad is listening to our conversation, hiding deep under his bedcovers in preparation for his mother's volcanic eruption of some sort.

However, no eruption ensued, not even short, clipped answers; rather, she told me more in that next ten minutes than Thad had heard in his whole twenty-four years of life. She seemed to enjoy talking about this wonderful man who gave her three beautiful children to love and who loved her. She considered their children a wonderful tribute to the love they shared.

We laugh about it now: how a young, outspoken Italian girl could come into a quiet German family and bring out so much information for such a good cause. This is strange because I usually bring havoc!

Surviving and Thriving

Don't let fear prevent you from getting the knowledge and information that may save your life one day.

Prayer

We often worry about what to say and what not to say, Lord. So rather than risk being wrong, we miss opportunities to draw ourselves closer, to learn from those who have the knowledge that can alter our lives. Help us to know when to speak with words and when to speak with silence.

· · ·

7-5. MEDICAL RECORD-KEEPING—IT COULD SAVE YOUR LIFE

An intelligent heart squires knowledge, and the ear of the wise seeks knowledge.

Proverbs 18:5 (ESV)

When I was twenty years old, completing the doctor's intake forms was a breeze. I didn't have much to record except age, weight, and a few childhood diseases—all of which were easy to recall. Fast-forward fifty years, and I am lucky I can remember my address, let alone all the medical issues I have survived. My mind has grown confused from walking the tightrope of being a wife, mother, sister, aunt, employee…oh, and of being menopausal.

Another factor is that my medical records are located in various places, such as the offices of my current family physician (I have had several), an orthopedic physician, two gynecologists, two dermatologists, a radiation specialist, several surgeons, an oncologist, a cardiologist, and a chiropractor, as well as two local hospitals and one out-of-state hospital. I'm having a power surge just thinking about all the doctors I have seen! Each has various pieces of information that make up my medical history, whether it's allergies, test results, surgeries, childhood illnesses, or shots.

When a medical emergency arises, it is critical that you have all your medical records, or those of a loved one, in one place where they are easily accessible. What if your loved one is deathly allergic to a certain type of medication, but you can't remember which one? When the EMTs arrive is not the time to scramble around looking for medical records. Take care of this extremely important task now so you will be ready in the event of an emergency.

How do you keep track of all the dates, tests, and medical events in your life? Do you write them on sticky notes? Do you have notes scribbled illegibly on bills from doctors, or do you have a cheat sheet? Maybe you do none of the above and just bury your head in the sand and hope the doctor can figure it out by the bumps, scars, and current symptoms. The federal mandate to require electronic medical records (EMR) across health-care systems will alleviate this problem, but many doctors' offices lag behind in converting all their paper records to EMR.

Why is it important for patients to keep medical records? First, to organize the many ever-changing, ever-evolving facets of medical care and second, to empower *you*, the patient. When you are faced with an illness, you often feel helpless and at the mercy of the health-care system.

One way to override feelings of helplessness is to gain knowledge. Learning all you can about your body and options is imperative to arming yourself against illness and making your way back to good health. It is more import-

---

One way to override feelings of helplessness is to gain knowledge

---

ant than ever that you have the knowledge to care for your own well-being. Medical record-keeping is *not* meant to replace a physician's records but is meant to assist you and your health-care professional. By keeping your medical records in one central and organized area, you and your physician can use the information to streamline your care.

Because of a lack of space, many hospitals and offices keep records for a limited amount of time. For example, in my case, the slides taken at my breast biopsy will be kept for only three years (check with your physician and hospital to find out how long they store records). Should I have a recurrence, say, in ten years, the surgeon would not have the advantage of comparing the prior tumor slides with the current ones. However, having this information could greatly aid in the treatment of the second tumor.

Even the prophets wrote the history they were living in. Why not you? Several methods of record-keeping are available to you. You may choose to keep the records yourself or enlist the help of services designed to store your files on the Internet for you. Whatever system you choose, use it!

Taking an active part in the record-keeping of your medical history benefits both you and the physician. It educates you in the process of your healing. It allows you the ability to study the findings calmly, in your own environment, where you can formulate possible questions for your physician. Having your questions answered is a big step to feeling empowered in making medical decisions that are suitable and appropriate for you. With your questions answered, the doctor will find a calmer, more compliant patient, one who is knowledgeable and capable of making a decision that both you and your physician can live with.

Surviving and Thriving

Compiling all your medical history into one location gives you the big picture of your health, which will assist your physician in providing you with better care, and better care means better health. I challenge you—I empower you—to keep records of every medical event, however insignificant it may seem. That insignificant piece may be the one that saves your life.

Prayer

God, You have entrusted us with honoring our bodies for Your glorification. Today I will begin to actively and patiently use all methods available to me, such as record-keeping, in pursuit of health and wellness. With good health, I will be more active in spreading Your Word and Your glory to others so they might see Your light shining through me.

. . .

IN CLOSING…

*I can do all things through Christ
who strengthens me.*

Philippians 4:13 (NKJV)

*For I am, the L*ORD *your God who takes hold of
your right hand and says; it is I who say to you,
"Do not fear, I will help you."*

Isaiah 41:13

Finally, I leave you with this thought: we know how truly connected the mind and body are to good health. Attitude is half the battle. As you face a medical challenge, arm yourself with resources such as health information materials, professional people, loved ones, and friends. Take care of all your needs—spiritual, physical, and mental. Listen to your body, and listen to your soul.

I challenge you to view your illness(es) as an opportunity for learning, growing, seeing yourself empowered by the knowledge you gain, and growing in Christ's love. Top that list by keeping Christ close. Fear is one of our biggest illnesses, but we have the best prescription ever: God's Word—the Bible.

The Bible shows us how those who have gone before us traversed those difficult times, were paralyzed with fear, but were strengthened by God's promise. Exodus 33:14 tells us, "My presence will go with you, and I will give you rest." In Genesis 26:24, God promises us, "Do not be afraid, for I am with you." Therefore, no matter how busy, stressed, angry, tired, or frustrated you are, arm yourself with faith. Arm yourself with all the tools that God has given you as you traverse the medical maze on your way to eternity.

Prayer

I would like to end with Paul's prayer to the Ephesians:

> *I pray that out of his glorious riches he may strengthen you with power through his Spirit in your inner being, so that Christ may dwell in your hearts through faith. And I pray that you, being rooted and established in love, may have power, together with all the Lord's holy people, to grasp how wide and long and high and deep is the love of Christ, and to know this love that surpasses knowledge—that you may be filled to the measure of all the fullness of God (Eph. 3:16–19).*

Dear Reader,

Thank you for taking the time to read *Surviving Medical Mayhem*. I pray that my stories, along with God's words, provided you with a "peace that surpasses all understanding." I thank you for the opportunity to make a difference.

Loretta Schoen

And the peace of God, which transcends all understanding, will guard your hearts and your minds in Christ Jesus.

Philippians 4:7

ABOUT THE AUTHOR

Loretta Schoen is a survivor of medical mayhem. God has been providing Loretta Schoen with firsthand life experiences so that she might share with others who are traversing or have traversed these same roads of medical adversity. Through the plethora of medical events in her life and in the lives of those around her, Loretta has been gaining medical knowledge and applying it to her passion: helping others turn from being stressed to feeling blessed. Her writing is candid, peppered with humor, and heavily salted with God's Word to sustain the journey.

Loretta was born in Glen Cove, New York, and she has lived in São Paolo, Brazil; Rome, Italy; and North Carolina. She currently resides in Central Florida with her husband of forty-three years in what she affectionately calls "The Schoen Assisted-Living Facility." Loretta has a passion for music, traveling, working with abused animals, spending time with her daughter and son-in-love, and being "Nana" to her grandsons, Aiden and Ryker.

Ten of her stories have been published in five different volumes of *Chicken Soup for the Soul.*

Surviving Medical Mayhem
Laughing When It Hurts

www.lorettaschoen.com

If you're a fan of this book, will you help me spread the word?

There are several ways you can help me get the word out about the message of this book…

- Post a 5-Star review on Amazon.

- Write about the book on your Facebook, Twitter, Instagram – any social media you regularly use!

- If you blog, consider referencing the book, or publishing an excerpt from the book with a link back to my website. You have my permission to do this as long as you provide proper credit and backlinks.

- Recommend the book to friends – word of mouth is still the most effective form of advertising.

- Purchase additional copies to give away as gifts.

I know you'll find this hard to believe but I like to talk! So if you'd like me to speak to your group, by all means, reach out to me. I want to bring encouragement, help and hope to anyone who may be wrestling with their own version of "medical mayhem."

The best way to connect with me is by: Loretta@lorettaschoen.com

NOTES